ALICE ON THE LINE

T0359427

Doris Blackwell
Douglas Lockwood

NEW
HOLLAND

Published in Australia by New Holland Publishers
Sydney

Level 1, 178 Fox Valley Road, Wahroonga, NSW 2076, Australia

newhollandpublishers.com

First published by Rigby Publishers 1975
Reprinted by Seal Books edition 1974, 1976, 1978, 1980, 1981
Reprinted by Lansdowne Publishing Pty Ltd 1996
Reprinted by New Holland Publishers in 2001, 2008, 2010, 2018, 2021, 2022, 2024

A record of this book is held at the National Library of Australia.

ISBN 9781741108033

Managing Director: Fiona Schultz
Production Director: Arlene Gippert
Cover Design: Hayley Norman
Printed in China

10 9 8

Keep up with New Holland Publishers:
 NewHollandPublishers
 @newhollandpublishers

To the memory of my parents,
without whose loving
and cheerful common sense
our childhood at Alice Springs at the
turn of the century
would not have been so happy.

DORIS BRADSHAW BLACKWELL

AUTHOR'S NOTE

These pages from the past would not have been possible if I had had to depend entirely on my own memory.

More than sixty years have passed since I was taken to Alice Springs in a horsedrawn buggy and so have many of my contemporaries.

Having been persuaded to leave a record of life on the old telegraph stations in Central Australia, I must acknowledge my gratitude to friends who have willingly hunted through papers and letters and their own memories.

I am especially indebted to Mr L. B. Spicer, who joined the telegraph station staff at Alice Springs in 1905, and stayed on there and at Barrow Creek for several years after we left.

He responded generously to many an S O S by calling on his own superior memory to help fill blank spaces in mine. He also gave me access to letters written to his sister, which she wisely preserved.

Doris Bradshaw Blackwell

Kingswood, S.A.
1965

CONTENTS

ILLUSTRATIONS

Chapter One

TO ALICE WITH EASE

SOMETHING VERY MYSTERIOUS INDEED WAS going on in our home. For days there had been intriguing scraps of conversation in muttered undertones. Confidential talks between my mother and father had become much more frequent than usual. Even to an eight-year-old girl who could not yet claim to be blessed by woman's intuition there was nevertheless an unmistakable atmosphere of Something Doing.

But what? What could it be that my parents were so careful to keep from me? What could possibly have come into their lives that I shouldn't know about? A new baby? A death in the family? No, I felt it was neither of these.

How infuriating it was, and how frustrating to be told constantly, "Now run along, Doris, there's a good girl." And then doors would be shut to me and voices lowered and I couldn't get a clue of any kind as to what might be Up.

I was then of an inquiring and curious nature. To me, puzzles were for unravelling and mysteries for solving. Now here was one in the heart of my own home and I couldn't work it out. To a young girl who dearly loved to be "in" on things, to be privy to all the family gossip, this deliberate exclusion was annoying in the extreme. My school studies suffered and I lay awake at night searching for the explanation, the revelation that would not come. I fretted until I dropped unhappily asleep, only to resume the quest from the moment I wakened. But there was never a single tangible clue on which I could put my finger and never an unguarded word from my parents which might have betrayed them.

Then in due time I was told all about it and wondered why I had been expecting calamity when in fact it was merely a bombshell.

We were going to Alice Springs!

In these days of comfortable trains and jet air travel a visit to Central Australia might not seem remarkable. The train trip in air-conditioned sleeping carriages is completed in two days. By flying, it is possible to be in Alice Springs just three hours after leaving Adelaide. Things were very different for me and my family, for when I was eight we were still in the nineteenth century. To be sure, the year was 1899, but I have always taken smug satisfaction in announcing it. It sounds so much more impressive than 1900, the beginning of the century of the horseless carriage, the radio, aeroplanes, earth satellites, and other miracles we had never imagined.

The news of our impending departure came at a time when the Adelaide streets had horse-drawn trams and the narrow-gauge railway to the north terminated at Oodnadatta, 688 miles away—but still more than 300 miles short of our destination. I was pleasantly excited at the prospect of having to drive in a buggy over this last long distance, especially when I realized that for more than a week we would camp each night beside our sandy track.

Within a few days, however, anticipation gave place to trepidation.

When I told my friends at the Church school in Halifax Street of the great adventure ahead of me I was bursting with importance. That bubble was soon pricked because none of them had ever heard of Alice Springs. It had been in existence for only thirty years and, of course, hadn't yet been blessed with a dot and a name on the maps in our geography books. I suffered a certain loss of face to be leaving the State's beautiful and growing capital city for a place that didn't yet exist—if the cartographers were to be believed.

"Go on, show us Alice Springs on the map!" My friends wanted proof.

I was upset and disappointed yet put on the defensive by this, to me, churlish attitude.

"I can't show it to you on the map because it's too new," I said. "It's really just been discovered. These maps they're old... they wouldn't even know about Alice Springs."

"But how do you know it's there?"

"I know...well, because I just know, that's all."

This illogicality was no proof at all and the torments continued to the point at which I might have burst into tears. Fortunately, I had an inspiration instead.

"I know it's there because my father is going to send all the telegrams and cables to Adelaide from Darwin, and even from London. We're going to live in a big house and we'll have horses to ride, and there'll be lots of kangaroos ..."

"And wild blackfellows" one boy said.

My eyes must have flickered with fright, for he seized the advantage with the sadistic glee of young boys everywhere.

"Yes, I've heard of people going up there and I'm sorry for them," he said. "You never hear of them again."

"Why?" It was a question I shouldn't have asked if I wanted to sleep at night, but I had to know the answer.

"They get eaten by the blacks, that's why," he said.

I saw the huge satisfaction spread over his face at what was obviously wide-eyed fear in mine, and then he turned the knife.

"Sometimes they find the bones. Sometimes they don't. People have even been known to escape the blacks, but those that do are always eaten by wild animals,"

He let me absorb this horrifying information for a short while and then asked: "Have you ever heard of anyone returning from Alice Springs? Do you know of anyone who has been there and come back?" There was an awful finality about the emphasis on his last two words.

I had to admit that I knew of nobody who had been to Alice Springs and returned to Adelaide. Before I could tell him that was because I didn't know anyone who had even been there, he said: "That's why. They all get eaten." And for the rest of the day, until I could get home to my mother and be reassured, he left me to the torment of my thoughts.

My father was Thomas Andrew Bradshaw, then aged forty. He had been born in England and migrated with his parents to the Portland district in Victoria when he was still a child. In his youth he joined the `Telegraph Office in Portland. In 1878, aged nineteen, he went to Adelaide and took a position with the Telegraph Department at the General Post Office. He became an expert telegraphist, a man who read Morse code with his ears and "spoke" it with his fingers as though it were his mother-tongue.

The horse-drawn trams did not run after dark, probably because the horses were not fitted with headlights, so my father had to walk to work each night from our home in Halifax Street. We were quite close to the city and he didn't seem to mind; indeed, except on cold winter nights, I imagine that he welcomed the opportunity for exercise that was otherwise denied him by the demands of his sedentary occupation.

We must have moved to the small villa-fronted stone house in Halifax Street, identical with several others, when I was three or four years old. My brother, Mort, was then a baby. My sister Consie and my younger brother Jack were both born there, Consie in 1896 and Jack in 1897.

My recollections of that period are dim, especially as my life was soon so completely transformed that stronger memories have pushed them into the background. But I do remember the broad acres of natural parklands surrounding the inner city and separating it from the infant suburbs. I remember being taken there to romp in a rural setting that might have been many miles away in the bush, an impression heightened by the fact that in those days we were free of the noise of internal combustion engines, the imperious honking of horns, and the clangorous cacophony of a modern city.

Today our street lights are flashed on when an invisible man presses a switch in some unfamiliar power station. But the lamp-lighter who came down Halifax Street at dusk every evening was a friend of ours. We envied him. He rode a bicycle and we always greeted each other. He carried a long stick with a hook on the end with which he pulled a chain perhaps fifteen feet above the pavement—and, lo, there was light. We knew that our gas-lamps were his personal responsibility and we trusted him. But who is responsible now for such important matters, and whom do we trust? A man, no doubt, who does it all by remote control; who sits behind a desk by a master panel and makes hundreds of lights come on at once. Does he know they are on? Can he see them? Has he ever seen any of them alight? I wonder does he know that his job was once done by artisans who stopped beneath each pole to make sure the lamp was burning before moving on to the next...ensuring that Thomas Bradshaw, as he walked home after a night filled with the dots and dashes of Morse code, wouldn't trip on the cobbles and kerbs of Halifax Street.

We had a few simple diversions. I'm afraid that one of these was at the expense of a Chinese merchant who frequently came shuffling down our street with two square boxes suspended from a shoulder yoke. He always had a crowd of children running after him. Unlike the Bradshaws, who endeavoured to look sweet and innocent, many of them had apparently not heard the legend that he would chase and do something dreadful to anyone who shouted, as they often did: "Ching Chong Chinaman, all so velly nice." Inside the boxes were shelves filled with drapery and haberdashery which he opened for the housewives to consider and buy. I will always remember how those heavy boxes creaked and swayed when he lifted them on his yoke and resumed jog-trotting along the street, frequently without making a sale. I felt deeply sorry for him.

St John's Church of England, our parish church, was quite near our home. It was fashionable for weddings and we spent many happy hours there waiting for brides to emerge and be pelted with rice we begged from our mothers. Confetti was unknown. Our substitute for empty cans tied behind today's bridal limousines were old shoes tied to a horse-drawn carriage.

Because we lived so close to a church we also saw more than our share of funerals, with everything so black and sombre: black hearses drawn by black horses with black plumes nodding from their black manes; undertakers, black clad, with black crepe streamers flying from their black silk hats; widows in black weeds, with black-pleated Mary Tudor caps and black streamers, and even handkerchiefs edged in black. It was not to be long before I discovered that black people—the aborigines we were soon to see—used white for their mourning.

The ice-cream man came down our street. What a treat today's children miss in not having him as we did. They buy their chocolate-coated sticks, their double-headers, their neapolitans, and a dozen flavours from the antiseptic deep-freeze at the corner shop. But our man came in a cart with bells tinkling from a pony's mane. His ice-cream wasn't made in aluminium vats, but in a wooden churn packed with ice and salt which he wound himself until he had a confection fit for the angels. And all for one penny! There was an organ grinder with a red-capped monkey which collected pennies; a bottle-and-rag man, and another who drove slowly around the streets warbling in a sweet tenor that we might buy from him "garden 'oney."

Penny-farthing bicycles were occasionally ridden down our street, but when family friends, Mr and Mrs Butler, rode to our place from Norwood on conventional bicycles the sight was so unusual that residents ran to their front fences to get a better view.

Street musicians were everywhere. Later, at Alice Springs, my mother often sighed for the sound of Italians playing harps and violins on Glenelg jetty. She had to be satisfied with primitive songmen chanting corroboree lays to the clang of beating sticks! She also sighed for our neighbours, the seven members of the well-known Pank family of Adelaide, whose father taught each of them a musical instrument. Crowds gathered in the street outside their home while they rehearsed for concerts attended by people who arrived by horse-trams, in hansom cabs, gigs, and fourwheelers.

This, then, was the Adelaide I remembered and was to recall nostalgically almost daily during the next nine years in what might well have been a foreign land, Central Australia. Specifically, I was to miss the natural beauty of the parklands so nobly planned by Colonel Light as the city's lungs—its breathing place. In Alice Springs, to give it its due, there was never to be any lack of a place to breathe. On the contrary, the commodities we had most of were fresh air and open space. Yet the difference was marked, and remains so. Adelaide, surrounded by hills, is soft and verdant. Alice Springs, also surrounded by hills, is harsh and red.

The change came quickly and dramatically, as though an English family from the Sussex Downs or the dales of Dorset had suddenly found themselves transplanted in Saudi Arabia or North Africa. We left temperate greens for desert brown, grey cloud for blue sky, and came upon sand hills and spinifex and human beings whose skin was no longer uniformly white but most frequently black. Our trains, when we left the terminus at Oodnadatta, ceased to be iron horses and became lumbering camels—immense humped beasts whose padded feet carried them easily through the dunes and across the gibbers even though their backs were laden with quarter-ton loads.

There were times during the long hot summers when I dreamt of the sea, of ice-cream carts, of couch-grass lawns, and of tall eucalypts in the Mount Lofty Ranges. Along the banks of the Todd and the Charles rivers, hemmed in by the MacDonnell Ranges, there were ghostly gums that shone in the moonlight with a brilliance I had never seen. Yet the smell of drought was on this land. The dusty mulga, stunted and yellow, seemed perpetually thirsty. Other vast differences between our lives in these two places often occurred to me. But it is still true that when I left there, a woman of seventeen hankering for companionship and brighter lights, I did so as one who leaves an ancestral home. The tug at my heart, as we saw the last of the great Australian nothingness, was such that I knew I must never go back unless I was to be trapped for ever. The people who live in Alice Springs now will have difficulty in recognizing the place I describe, yet its enchantment then must have equalled that which draws tourists in thousands towards it today.

For some years my father had been in charge of the night staff at the Central Telegraph Office.

I have a fleeting memory of three rows of men in a large upstairs room in King William Street, each of them bent over keys or receivers, while an incomprehensible stutter of dah-dits filled the air and was somehow interpreted into English words and phrases by the skilled operators. How they could concentrate on the code coming from one machine while others near by were clattering just as noisily was always a mystery to me. I suppose that like people in crowded rooms they were able to tune in on the single conversation that interested them. In any case, they seldom hurried or appeared to be confused, but monitored their machines and hand-wrote hundreds of telegrams and cables which flowed through the office every day. None of them ever gave the slightest indication that they were affected by the endless accounts of joy and misery, of births and deaths, contained in their daily ration of private news.

Their work was onerous and continuous and demanded diligence of the most devoted kind. In those days every overseas cable message and every newspaper story from the other side of the world was transmitted from Darwin along the Overland Telegraph to Adelaide—one letter at a time in Morse code. Perhaps it isn't surprising, therefore, that three rows of operators working day and night were required to handle the traffic.

This, plus the strain of night duty and the added worry of supervising a staff, eventually began to affect my father's health. Finally he was prevailed upon to consult a doctor, who suggested a long sea trip. Although this was one of the basic prescriptions of the era, almost a stock-in-trade for the frock-coated doctors, it was scarcely soothing and practical advice to a civil servant, with a young family, who earned only five pounds a week.

Nevertheless, it must have been fortuitously apt, though ships of the desert and seas of spinifex were more likely than ocean travel in the future life of Thomas Bradshaw. As it happened, the position of officer-in-charge of the Alice Springs telegraph office was about to become vacant. Mr F. J. Gillen, whose name is perpetuated in mountains and books, was leaving the Centre after many years of faithful service. It must have impressed my father as an adequately remote place and quiet enough to soothe anyone's frayed nerves, for he applied for and was appointed to the position. Later I wondered if he realized that all Press and commercial cables would still pass through his hands in the Alice Springs repeater station.

Having been selected after weeks of delay, my father was required to go at once to take up his new position, leaving my mother to finalize their affairs, to engage a governess for the four young children, and to follow unescorted when that was possible. On a hot morning in March 1899, we said goodbye to him at Adelaide station. He was a short, stocky man with dark hair and brown eyes, a moustache, and a developing corpulence that the Aranda tribesmen dignified with the name "Adnutta."

At that time Alice Springs was literally in the back of beyond. To most Australians it remains there today, although quick travel is available for those who want it. As we waved goodbye I had little conception of the physical effort involved in reaching the centre of the continent at the turn of the century, but within two months I was to learn that the train which took my father to Oodnadatta, and was soon to take us, was named "The 'Ghan" because of its close association with Afghan camel teamsters who bridged the 300-mile gap between the terminus and Alice Springs. Camels! My goodness, I thought, perhaps there really were wild animals roaming in the desert.

My mother found rooms at Glenelg where we stayed until a cold dark morning in May when we caught the six-thirty suburban train to Adelaide for a rendezvous with adventure. It has often occurred to me since that for her this must have been a rather terrifying experience. She had the responsibility of four children under the age of eight. She was going into a country she had never seen and didn't understand. She knew with certainty that after several days in an uncomfortable train there would be a fortnight of desert travel by buggy. Her young brood would have to sleep with her beside the track with any amount of unknown but well imagined dangers—snakes, for instance—to disturb her sleep. She would know that at the end of the trip, a thousand miles from its beginning, the nearest doctor would then be at Oodnadatta or Marree, from three to five hundred miles away. There would be no hospital or nurse to ease the suffering of her children or the torment of her own mind if they became ill. I wonder did she realize that when serious accidents happened, as they sometimes did, my father would be required to act as locum tenens for an Adelaide doctor sitting in the Central Telegraph Office. He would tap out his Morse code message describing symptoms or explaining injuries. This would be translated to the doctor by the Adelaide operator, who would then send instructions back to Alice Springs. In that way, as I will later explain, he treated everything from blood poisoning to a broken hip, from sunstroke to malaria. I wasn't surprised to find among his effects a carefully preserved book in which were written the symptoms and treatment for dozens of diseases and illnesses likely to afflict us. But what kind of comfort was that for a young mother?

Only my mother's youth fitted her for such an adventure. She was thirty-three, as plump as mothers of four children should be, and with beautiful brown hair she had allowed to grow. She was courageous and practical, an able seamstress and a good cook. But beyond that she had no training which might help her overcome the difficulties she was about to face. On the contrary, her preparation for the desert consisted largely of a life on or by the sea. In fact, she was born there— on the liner Atalanta off the Cape of Good Hope on the way to Australia. To celebrate it, she was christened Atalanta Hope Allchurch.

In retrospect, it seems barely credible that a young mother should have been asked to go into the desert in these circumstances, without a minimum of medical training. Only two other white women lived in Alice Springs at that time; apart from them the nearest were at Hermannsburg Lutheran mission station, eighty miles and a two-day drive to the west. Yet my mother not only went to the Centre; for a time, at least, she seems to have enjoyed the experience, and there was seldom an emergency she couldn't cope with.

We were joined on the station platform on that first morning by Miss Bertha Easom, a slight fair girl in her early twenties whom Mother had engaged as a governess. She was of a bright disposition and not only eager to face the wilderness, barren as it might be of eligible young men, but apparently quite undismayed at the prospect of having four mischievous children in her charge. She was the first of a series of governesses who were my only teachers until I left Alice Springs at the age of seventeen. I would like to say here that I have always been grateful for their love, their skill, and their devotion to what I can imagine only as a thankless task. They must truly have been touched with the spirit of service, for I can think of no other reason why they should want to bury themselves in the dormant heartland away from their families and, presumably, any chance they might have of marrying. Nor could any of them have been attracted by the salary. My father's stipend was barely enough to support us, so that our teachers could never have got more than a few shillings a week.

These things may have worried my mother or Miss Easom, but they certainly did not worry me or my brothers and sister. To us, it was all simply a wonderful adventure. The train ride from Glenelg to the city had always enchanted us, but this time we would be in our carriages for three whole days. The aridity of coal dust, the hissing steam, the clang of bells, the cries of porters and guards, the rattle of trolleys with mountainous loads of mail and goods—these were all a part of the journey and as thrilling to us then as the more sophisticated preparations for travel today. What's more, we had greater leisure in which to enjoy it, and came to regard it as an extended picnic. None of this modern business of being confined in hermetically sealed air-conditioned carriages, antiseptic and almost noiseless. Ah, no! We travelled in a train in which the windows could be raised. We could lean out to watch the sleepers speeding by beneath us and hear the clatter of the wheels passing over the gaps in the rails. Nor were we kept there at night, tucked tightly in narrow bunks while we passed through country we couldn't see. Our train had no sleeping cars, so we stopped each night at a hotel—and the train waited for us until after breakfast next day. 1 still think that was a civilized way to do things.

After reaching Terowie, about a hundred and fifty miles north of Adelaide, we were put aboard the narrowgauge 'Ghan and remained in the same reserved carriage until Oodnadatta, where we arrived three days later. The compartment had a seat on either side for its entire length. This was a convenient arrangement as we could leave some of our toys and books and luggage there while we went to our hotel overnight—the first at Quorn, the second at Hergott Springs (renamed Marree during the first World War), and the third at Oodnadatta. Mrs Henderson, a superintendent's wife from up the track, and her little girl shared the carriage with us. Mrs Henderson had been born in Switzerland and spent the first part of her life surrounded by the beauty of the Swiss Alps and lakes. After we had left the Flinders Ranges behind and the country had begun to stretch out across the gibbers and salt bush I noticed she sighed frequently when she looked out of the window. At the age of eight those sighs meant little to me, but now I know exactly how she felt.

Mrs Henderson had been in the north for some years and was returning from a holiday in Adelaide. She had her own ideas about the correct way to treat the aborigines and the impropriety of certain forms of address. At one of our stops we came upon our first large group of them. I remember running back to the carriage with the news.

"Mother," I said excitedly, "there are some black ladies out there."

Mrs Henderson corrected me. "Natives, my dear. We don't call them ladies," she said.

Ladies or not, they were a great novelty to us and we seemed to be equally so to them and their wide-eyed children. The first of the early settlers were only then going to the Centre to take up land and the aborigines were still regarded more or less as savages, an attitude that has survived to this day with some Europeans. We found them docile, friendly people who were always glad to help us if they could. In the Petermann

Ranges, however, and in other outlying areas they were still hostile and dangerous, and explorers and land-seekers were frequently attacked.

It was a friendly, obliging sort of train, with a camaraderie between crew and passengers that would be almost unthinkable today. The locomotive was the centre of attraction for all the young boys (and some young girls, too), especially after one or two had been given rides on the foot- plate by the driver while he was shunting in and out of coaling depots. Occasionally one lucky boy was allowed to pull the cord which blew the whistle, an event he would talk about for days. They were shown the inside of the roaring furnace, and watched delightedly while the driver lifted the long handle which made steam enter the cylinders and drive the pistons that turned the wheels.

Even to a girl, there seemed to be something about a steam engine which is missing from the diesel and electric trains we have today. A Puffing Billy was almost alive. It hissed and snarled, grunted and whistled, and smoked like some monstrous human being. We came to regard ours as a friend almost as much as we did the driver and the firemen. These men, in their blue overalls with big sweat rags of cotton waste, were friends indeed. They made the trip a joy for us all. When we wanted a cup of tea, for instance, we simply took a teapot along to the driver at one of the frequent stopping places. He pressed a button and, presto! we had a potful of boiling water. Nor were they ever in a hurry; they didn't mind stopping for a yarn with passers-by, or waiting patiently for passengers who wandered off. If some were more than usually slow in returning to the train the driver would blow his whistle peremptorily, but never did he threaten to leave anyone behind. He knew none were travelling north for pleasure. Occasionally it happened that the driver and fireman were to blame for the delays. I remember one occasion when a lonely boundary rider was waiting at a siding for the train when we arrived. He had apparently ridden in from an isolated out-station because he was lonesome and "hungry for a yarn." After a prolonged conversation a shearer's head popped out of a window farther along the train from us and he demanded, "Shake 'er -up, Bill; we'll never get there tonight!" After a few minutes, Bill "shook 'er up," and off we went.

On another occasion the train, travelling at about thirty miles an hour, was hailed by a horseman. The brakes were applied and we ground to a halt, apparently for no other reason than that the rider, who had been out of touch with civilization for many weeks, wanted to get the latest news.

He put his horse's head beside the footplate and lay stretched out along its mane while he and the driver swapped anecdotes...until the shearer's head appeared again and he said, "Eh, Bill, what d'ya reckon this is—Parliament or something? We'll never get to Oodna."

"What's your hurry?" Bill replied. "You'll wish you hadn't hurried once you get there and see the joint."

"But, Bill, we gotta get to Oodna tonight," the shearer repeated illogically.

"Listen, mate," Bill said, "we don't gotta do nothing of the kind. This is a fortnightly service, ain't it? Well, I've got a week to get there and a week to get back, and at present we've got two full days to play with. I don't care if we don't get there till Ash Wednesday...and I wouldn't care if we didn't get there at all."

Nevertheless, Bill's good nature got the better of him and within quarter of an hour he blew the whistle and we were off again.

" 'Bout time, too," the shearer growled. "The rate this thing's going we'll never get to Oodna."

We, too, were glad to be moving again. Bill the driver may not have been in a hurry, but for us the novelty of the barren countryside and the noise and discomfort of the train had long ago ceased to be exciting. It was late each night before we got to bed and we were up just as soon as Bill sounded reveille on the locomotive's whistle. Moreover, we carried only enough food for each day's journey—bread, tinned meat, biscuits, and fruit which we ate in the carriage as the train rolled along. In 1899 the 'Ghan was still many years from the day when white-coated stewards would serve four-course meals in well-appointed dining cars. And so it was without regret that we saw Algebuckina, Mount Dutton, and finally Allandale sidings disappear behind us as we wound around the gibbers on a long slow curve which took us down across the Neales and into the Oodnadatta basin.

Chapter Two

THANKS FOR THE BUGGY RIDE

OODNADATTA AT THE TURN OF THE CENTURY...
Desolation was everywhere. The south-east trade winds, bitterly cold, flicked up dust and pebbles and made life miserable. I discovered what Bill the driver had meant when he told the shearer that his haste was unwarranted. A handful of galvanized iron buildings represented the State's most northerly town—the biggest centre of habitation, indeed, between Port Augusta and Port Darwin on the other side of the continent.

It existed because it was the terminus of the railway and supplied a few outlying cattle stations, notably Todrnorden, Macumba, Dalhousie, and Blood's Creek. The desert encroached on all sides, apparently limitless, the only street extending into a vista of nothing that went on to the horizon. The quaint low-roofed hotel, by city standards, was not more than a "room on the route"; but in these surroundings it was the hub of all social life and saw a prodigious amount of beer drinking.

There was a small store, a major part of whose stock consisted of saddlery for horses and camels. Yes, camels. I had seen them grazing on the outskirts of the town, their grotesque heads dwarfed by immense bodies, and I knew that they were used to carry the freight from our train over the remaining three hundred miles of unmade track to Alice Springs. I saw half a dozen houses, one occupied by an itinerant doctor. When I think back now, I am surprised that the area had a doctor at all; the population couldn't have been more than one hundred, most of them hardy bushmen who seldom fell ill and wouldn't go to a doctor if they did. A Doctor Shanahan, who served Oodnadatta from farther south, had a buggy drawn by small Timor ponies, and he drove to Alice Springs once during our stay there, when typhoid fever broke out on the goldfield at Winnecke.

I changed my city frock for a starched white pinafore to look as appropriately dressed as possible for my father, who had driven down from Alice Springs to meet us. Next morning he took us all for a walk around the town, to inspect the shop, the private homes, which seemed naked without gardens (for the town was short of water), and the herds of goats wandering aimlessly around and subsisting on what they could find. 1 have been told that goats will eat anything and can live on the smell of an oily rag, but at Oodnadatta they apparently kept themselves alive on gibbers and sand.

My clearest recollection of that morning walk is of a yard surrounded by a high fence made of saplings with a central post supporting a thatched roof. Chained to the post by their wrists were six or seven natives, who sat on the ground with their feet towards us. I have never forgotten the horror of seeing human beings thus chained, but worse still was the sight of their bleeding and swollen feet. They stared dumbly at us, perhaps aware that there was nothing we could do to alleviate their suffering. We were told that they had been caught spearing cattle on one of the big station properties in the Centre and were on their way to Port Augusta gaol to serve long prison sentences. A police trooper with two aboriginal trackers, all mounted, had brought the poor creatures from Alice Springs. The prisoners, chained together by their wrists, and at night by their ankles as well, had walked every step of more than three hundred miles to the railhead. In the years that followed I saw many natives in chains, but I was no less revolted on subsequent occasions than I was at Oodnadatta with this first glimpse of man's bestiality to man. The chaining of human beings, even to my young mind, seemed depraved and sadistic. Yet it was so commonplace that I cannot recall ever having seen aboriginal prisoners who were not in chains. Once or twice I saw men who had walked so far in lawful custody that they had no skin left on the soles of their feet.

I do not imagine that detention in Port Augusta gaol acted as the slightest deterrent in stopping the spearing of cattle, unless that was achieved by the extreme cruelty of the forced marches. To primitive aborigines, life in gaol must have represented the acme of comfort. They would be given regular meals, shelter from the cold winds, and blankets to sleep in— experiences which may even have produced a halo of romance when they returned to their tribes and told the stories of what they had seen and done.

This was early preparation for the crudity of life as I was often to see it henceforth. The doleful sight in that Oodnadatta yard may have helped lessen my anguish in the future; at least it prevented my lapsing into a state of shock and having to be given smelling salts after some of the stories we heard. One of these, related quite matter-of-factly by a policeman who had been stationed north of Alice Springs, revealed that when they were sent to catch and punish natives accused of spearing cattle they used piccaninnies for target practice. I came very close to fainting when that story was told.

Not all the men in Central Australia were cruel or even unkind to the natives. There were a few shining exceptions. But I was to know instances of such injustice and cruelty that made me ashamed of my race.

My father had been in Oodnadatta for several days before our arrival, chiefly to rest the horses for the return trip, heavily laden, through the fearful sandhills. He had already been travelling for ten days, and would cover a total of more than six hundred miles by buggy so that his family might have the comfort of his presence during their first drive into the Never-Never. As well as the telegraph station buggy, he brought a buckboard; this was a lower vehicle, with a single seat near the front and a long flat tray for luggage. He was accompanied by a wonderful Englishman named George Hablett, a casual station worker who stayed with the telegraph staff at Alice Springs for thirty-three years and said when he left, "I wouldn't have taken the job if I'd known it wasn't permanent." Also in the party was Bob Crann, who later died of thirst in the desert.

My first view of the buggy and buckboard wasn't at all reassuring. We had been for three days in a railway carriage where we had plenty of room to move around. Now we were to be eighteen days in an open buggy, running across gibbers and sand and through creeks on iron-tyred wooden wheels. We would have no protection from sun or rain and no room at all to move; in any case, to have done so while the buggy was in motion was prohibited by my father in case we fell off in the rough going.

The buggy was designed to seat five people, but it carried seven. Mother sat in the front seat with Jack, my eighteen-month-old brother, and the driver. Miss Easom, Mort, Consie, and I were on the rear seat. Waterbags and frying pans, gridirons and quartpots were hung underneath, clattering about like a drum and steel band. Our trunks, bags and boxes of food, swags, blankets, shovels, spare harness—and my father—were carried on the buckboard. By the time thirty reserve horses and two aboriginal helpers joined the convoy we must have looked like a poor man's edition of Wirth's Circus.

Our buggy was drawn by five sturdy horses—they had to be strong to be chosen for the task—and the buckboard by four. There were also a number of packhorses, loaded with the men's swags and the tent, which followed behind the wheeled vehicles. They never tried to run away. Alice Springs was their home country and they were keen to return there. I hadn't yet seen that part of the world, but I didn't blame them for so obviously wanting to leave the scant pastures around Oodnadatta.

The teams were changed each day at noon; even so, the journey was a gruelling test for the horses. No fodder was ever carried; they were hobbled and turned loose at night to find what feed they could, but that was always scarce around the wells where we camped because so many others had been there before them. Although hobbled, they sometimes wandered almost half-way back to our last camp during the night, giving the aborigines many extra miles to cover to round them up and make a start possible next morning. The wells were spaced about thirty miles apart, a fair day's journey in the heavy going. Horses taken on the track were given a long spell beforehand, and only those in the best condition were chosen. Nevertheless, some nearly always "knocked up" and had to be abandoned. All looked wretched at the end of the journey, especially in the poor seasons.

To an eight-year-old girl these were matters of small importance, if they were considered at all. This was by far the greatest adventure of my young life and I was determined to enjoy every phase of it. If my own daughter, when she was eight, had been required to drive from Oodnadatta to Alice Springs in a buggy I'd have been extremely concerned. I had no such concern for myself. I was with my parents and several practical men who understood the desert and its whims—or so I believed. In any case, I felt secure enough on my seat, and looked forward to the novelty of sleeping on the ground through the nights to come.

"Giddap! Gee orff! Move on there, Toby! Come on now, come on, come on!"

At last we were all aboard for the buggy ride; the drivers had taken up their reins and begun flicking them, pulling on the bits of the leaders to bring them to an awareness of the task ahead; and the verbal orders began—to continue almost incessantly until we reached Alice Springs. This was one of the charms of early travel: the communication between the driver and his horsepower which disappeared with the advent of internal combustion engines.

The buggies began to roll, slowly at first, until the teams settled down and they could be encouraged or goaded into a trot when the track permitted it. We bounced over gibbers and other protrusions; the harness creaked and flapped and the buggies rattled; collars and harries bounced on the necks of the sturdy beasts; soon they became warm and thereafter we had the smell of sweating horses constantly in our nostrils, a harsh animal smell that I've remembered all my life.

I looked back and saw Oodnadatta dancing in a mirage—white painted buildings seemingly suspended above the ground where the haze separated them from it. Next time I looked it was gone, and so was Oodnadatta, and I wasn't sorry. Surrounding us now for as far as one could see there was absolutely nothing that was man-made. The flat floor of an ugly desert stretched out on all sides until it disappeared where the earth met the cloudless sky. I had a Christian upbringing and have believed all my life in a Creator; yet, to say the least of it, the Oodnadatta country impressed me as being among the less lovely works of the Supreme Architect.

I imagined that because the country had grown progressively poorer as we got farther north, it would become poorer still as we travelled. There was nothing to suggest an end to the unbroken basin of gibbers and sand and occasional stunted bushes. I had no reason to believe that Alice Springs would not be like this, so I wondered how I was going to accustom myself to living in such desolation. I asked my father about it.

"Father, is Alice Springs as deserty as this?"

"Oh, no, Doris," he said. "It's a beautiful place, set inside a range of mountains, with a river bed running through it, and big ghost gums growing everywhere. You'll like it." He had to shout to make himself heard from the buckboard, but this gave his words an emphasis that was reassuring. I ceased to worry.

On and on we went, first with the sun on our right, then overhead, and eventually dropping down in the western sky. But the only shadows it made were those of us, our horses, our buggies, and the telegraph poles. We were passing through a land where no shadows are, a land where the sun might have been deprived of its power of reflection, so little was there to interrupt the stark flatness of the landscape.

On and on, walking and trotting, the wooden spokes casting moving images, the sand adhering to the iron tyres until halfway up the wheel, there to curl over and be taken down by gravity in a spiral of flying drift that never failed to fascinate me. This is also one of the most vivid memories of my sister Consie, then aged three.

On and on we drove, with the strain and creak of harness, and the white foam on flanks and withers being beaten by the traces and leather collars.

In all that vast land there was not one fence, or any track other than the one we used. But we knew that civilization was ahead of us, for we followed the slender iron poles supporting the two wires of the Overland Telegraph line—the reason for our journey. The line stretched ahead interminably, so far that we could not distinguish the poles from one another where they ran into the horizon. Beside the line we often saw old wooden poles, the originals put there twenty-seven years earlier and replaced when the voracious appetite of the white ants was discovered. There was one pole every seventy yards—about fifteen thousand of them between Adelaide and Alice Springs.

The novelty of buggy travel soon wore off—probably on that first day—and I had time to reflect upon the fact that except for government parsimony we might have made the entire journey by train, and gone on to Darwin if we had wished. In 1896 offers had been made to the South Australian Government, on behalf of various syndicates, to build a railway connecting Oodnadatta with the North Australia railway terminus at Pine Creek, only a hundred and fifty miles south of Darwin. The Government refused to accept any of the offers because they were based on the land grant system, although that was known to have succeeded in other countries. Driving through this country in a buggy, one was at a complete loss to understand why people foolish enough to want to waste money on trying to develop the desert, and build a railway to boot, should be discouraged. Paradoxically, by 1902 the Government had changed its mind to such an extent that it offered land grants around the world to big corporations which might have been interested in the proposal. More than a thousand miles of 3 ft. 6 in. track was to be built for a bonus of eighty million acres of freehold land, plus the right to operate a train service. Companies were found to be interested, and a contract with one of them was brought to signing point. But the scheme collapsed at the last minute because the fledging Federal government had placed restrictions on the employment of coloured labour. Hence, when we left Alice Springs in 1908, we still had to travel by buggy.

Our first night's camp was at a creek called the Swallow, which took the definite article like the Finke, the Alice, the Tennant, and so many other places in the north. But that's about all it did have! I remember that by the end of the first day I had become disenchanted with life in the outback as long as it had to do with buggy travel. I don't think I ever got used to these long slow trips, although we made several of them.

The Swallow was a place that did not exist on any map, for which the cartographers could scarcely be blamed, and

Myself when young... what the fashionable teenager wore in 1906

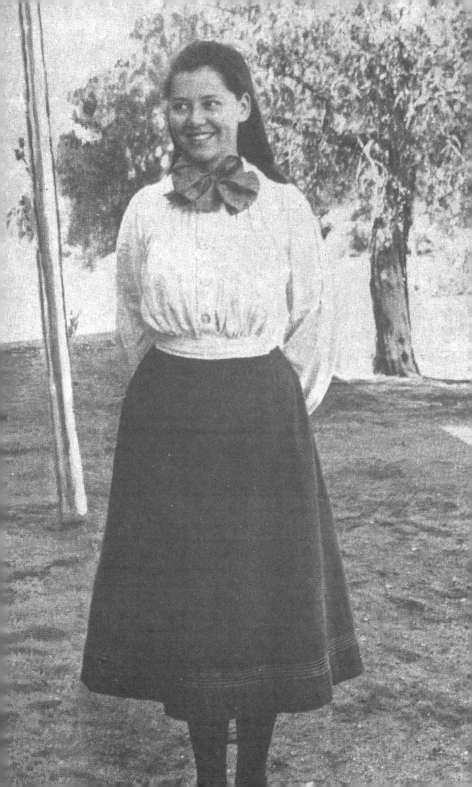

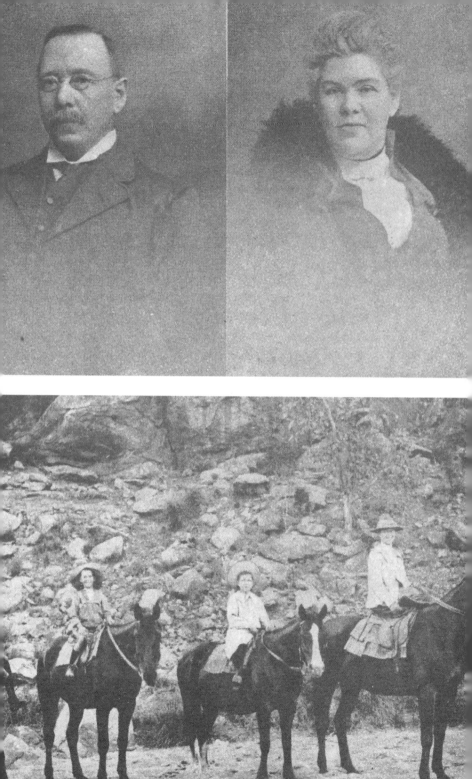

I doubt if it has been dignified with that importance today. I imagine we stopped there, and where we did on succeeding nights, because it was a comparatively good feeding place for the horses. They were always the prime consideration; we could be so tired that sitting upright on the armless buggy seats was scarcely possible, but we had to go on until we found water and horse feed.

Further realities of life in the "bush"—what a misnomer that was—were to catch up with me that night. After eight years of the comfort of kapok mattresses and feather pillows I found that my bed, until we reached Alice Springs, was to be a blanket-roll on the ground. How hard it was! Poets have found beauty and authors romance in swag-rolls, starlit heavens, sputtering billycans on campfires; and yarning by night in the soft light, but to me it all amounted to nothing more than sheer discomfort.

These night camps meant extremely hard work for the men, who could not rest until horses had been unharnessed, watered, and hobbled, the bedding and food unloaded, saplings cut to support the tent, a campfire made, and meals prepared. In the morning, the procedure was reversed. My mother always remembered the first camp at the Swallow because there she lost a brooch given to her as a farewell present. I remembered it because I had ceased to be enchanted and was frankly bored. The ground was hard and cold and I did not sleep well. I was probably worried about snakes and spiders and other dreadful forms of life that might decide to share the warmth of my swag.

Furthermore, the food was horrible—different, yes, but still horrible! Our menu consisted of salt beef and Oodnadatta bread, which soon became rock-hard. Jack, the baby, must

My father, Thomas A. Bradshaw, and my mother.
Photographed in 1916
From left: Mortimer, Jack, Consie, and myself

have lived almost exclusively on tinned milk; neither his teeth nor his digestion would have been able to cope with the tough meat. The tinned butter soon became sickly oil, and how I hated the tucker box!

It was an ingenious box, really, full of small compartments specially designed for the shapes and sizes of various canned and packaged foods. Each compartment had a leather lid held by a strap to keep things in place during the buffeting on the track, but it gave off an odour that I could recognize blindfold more than sixty years later. There was a mingling of pepper and pickles, salt beef and greasy calico bags, condensed milk and fat, stale bread and melted butter—all of it liberally coated with red dust and powdered sand which gritted on the teeth and made me shudder.

One day as we drove along a very rough part of the road known as Hell's Gates the tucker box fell off the buckboard. If we could have survived without it, I'd have left it there. This minor accident made a brief diversion in the monotony of the day's travel but poor Jack had to suffer for it. His milk bottle was the only casualty; it flew out and shattered in a thousand pieces. Anyhow, it was time he grew up and this was as good an opportunity as any for him to start; he philosophically learnt to drink his condensed milk from a cup. I didn't adapt myself so well, and within twenty-four hours I couldn't eat the revolting food. Rather than fuss or pamper me, my parents left me alone. It hadn't taken them long to learn the lesson of the bush that if I was really ill other symptoms would soon be apparent; if not, nature would take over and my appetite return, as indeed it must have, for I remained in bouncing health.

I suppose it is natural that through the eyes of a city child, the desert, seen at such close quarters, would be overwhelming and perhaps a little frightening. The vastness and the never-ending immensity of it all baffled the imagination.

I'd had no conception that anything in the world, not even the sea, could be so literally "big." I had the comfort and constant reassurance of my parents, and yet there was something about the desert that I dreaded. I couldn't come to terms with it, and never did. My younger sister and brothers had toys to amuse them; in any case, they had not yet reached an impressionable age; but I was aware that my friends were beyond reach and would remain so for a longer time than I'd already lived. I was aware, too, that there would be nobody to take their place. We expected to be the only children of European blood in Alice Springs, and as the distance increased from my school chums in Halifax Street I was overcome by a great melancholy. This all changed, of course. I soon settled down to life in Alice Springs and look back upon my nine years there as a wonderful experience.

Nevertheless, I now wished that I could see something more than desert from the tent flap each morning. The land was absolutely flat, so much so that one might have been pardoned for questioning the geographers who said the earth was round. We travelled for hours and sometimes for days without seeing a landmark worthy of the name. When we did see one it was a matter for great excitement and a recitation of knowledge by the Old Hands. But if only there'd been a house or some other living soul to prove to me that this was inhabited country and not the surface of the moon my mind might have been set at rest. If another buggy had come rumbling along from the opposite direction I'd have known at once that ahead we would find others of our own species. I wanted to be convinced that I still lived in that place called "civilization," when all the signs were against it—and at that moment, miraculously, I had my proof.

I had been standing at the door of our tent, dressed in a warm serge frock, surveying the blighted scene. The southeast trade winds were blowing; feeling cold, I walked over to the campfire where breakfast was already being prepared. Somehow that morning did not seem quite as bad as its predecessors in spite of my yearning for confirmation of the existence of other life. The sun was rising, sending from clumps of spinifex long sharp shadows which would disappear later on. The air was exhilarating, putting an edge to the appetite of those who weren't revolted by the food. The wind was whistling through the leaves of a few desert oaks at the well—the first substantial trees we had seen in several days—pitching high to an animal wail before sighing and dying with the gusts. I had heard it during the night in the otherwise silent land and been glad that my mother and father were near.

As we squatted around the fire that morning my mother remembered the date—23rd May—the anniversary of my Aunt Emily's birthday. She had lived with us in Adelaide and felt our departure keenly.

It was not possible to telephone or, so it seemed, to send her any form of greeting. Nevertheless, Mother expressed the wish.

"I wish I could send her a telegram," she said.

I suppose I giggled at the preposterous idea that we might send a telegram from the middle of a desert. The nearest post office was at Oodnadatta, already several days' drive behind us, and we wouldn't see another until we reached Charlotte Waters.

"What are you laughing at?" my father asked. "Your mother wants to send a telegram—well, perhaps we can."

There was a twinkle in his eye, so I thought he was joking. My mother must have thought so too, for she hesitated when father told her to write out what she wanted to say.

"Go on," he said. "I'm serious. You want to send a telegram—all right, I'll send it for you. Emily will get it in Adelaide today."

Still doubting, my mother did as she was told. I stared incredulously as my father went to the packsaddles and returned with two peices of curved iron.

"Whatever are they?" I asked. "Are you going to send a telegram with those?"

"They will help," my father said. "They are really feet clamps. You will see how they're used in a moment."

He fitted them to his boots, and when mother's message was ready he shinned up the nearest telegraph pole with ridiculous ease. There he arranged the two wires so that they passed through a small transmitting instrument which could be carried in a pocket. In this way he tapped the line from the uninhabited wilderness and within a few moments my mother's greeting was in the Central Telegraph Office in Adelaide.

This was a demonstration of the kind of magical "civilized" thing that I needed, and I realized that, after all, we had not left the world I knew so very far behind.

In the early days of the O.T. Line, men who were in difficulties cut the wires to make sure of help, especially when they feared attack by hostile aborigines. At least one man is known to have died because he didn't realize that cutting the wires would save him. Another was so weak that he failed in his attempts to climb a pole and died at the base of it. By the time we went to Alice Springs wire-cutting was regarded as an extremely serious offence and the practice had ceased; it had caused too many interruptions to vital international communications to be used as a lifesaver for mere individuals. Moreover, line repair was a long and tedious job as the break had to be reached on horseback. A cut midway between Alice Springs and the next telegraph office at Barrow Creek meant a round trip of a hundred and seventy miles for someone, and perhaps two or three days' delay to the traffic.

Four or five days after our buggy ride began the Oodna-datta bread was finally pronounced uneatable even by the old bushmen. Slicing it was no longer possible because it was so hard that it powdered. George Hablett, co-driver and self-appointed cook, thereupon made a damper of flour, water, and baking soda in a camp oven. It tasted like a cross between rubber and plaster of Paris. but at least it was fresh, if not quite what an eight-year-old girl would want for a birthday party.

"Smother it in pickles, Doris," my father advised, "and then you won't taste anything else."

"Worcester sauce is the stuff for bush tucker," George Hablett said. "You put enough Worcester on your beef and damper and you wouldn't know you weren't eating turkey and ham that was smothered in Worcester. The taste of sauce gets a bit monotonous, but you forget that when you're roughing it."

Unfortunately, I disliked both pickles and Worcester sauce at that age and could not resort to such camouflage. Nor could I take George Hablett's advice to "try a bit of condensed milk on the damper." I doubted his claim that this made it taste like apple pie.

For my palate, George's "Johnny cakes" were a greater success. These were simply small dampers about the size of a yeast bun and cooked in the coals instead of in a camp oven.

When making Johnny cakes George took care that his fire was "just so." It had to be a certain size, with the coals glowing adequately. Then he placed the small cakes of dough in a nest in the fire, and shovelled hot coals over them.

"It's impossible to cook in the bush without a good shovel," he said. "A shovel out here is as important as a ladle in a kitchen."

I rather suspect that the Johnny cakes tasted better than the damper simply because the word "cakes" was in the name. I could almost imagine myself eating some of mother's cream sponge back home—but not quite. Inevitably, George's concoctions came from the coals under a thick crust of charcoal, ash, and burnt flour.

"Bit burnt, but not bad," George would say. Then, noticing my tentative bites, he'd take mine from me and file the charcoal off with a rasp used for shoeing horses.

George was what is known in the outback as "a bit of a character." He had been a seaman in the Royal Navy. When he spoke, apparently believing that he had to be heard by the entire fleet, he shouted at the top of his voice. He had smiling blue eyes set in a tanned, deeply lined face. In his ears he wore small gold earrings, like a gipsy, and on his head the cloth cap of the English working-classes. I don't think I ever saw him without it.

I first became aware of George's personality through his loud-hailer voice as soon as we stepped off the train at Oodnadatta. On being introduced to Miss Easom, who was young and attractive, George expressed his disappointment.

"What's the use of bringing only one?" he demanded. "You should've brought a cartload and let 'em loose up here."

I'm sure everyone in Oodnadatta that day heard him. He was credited with the ability, when singing sea-shanties in hotel parlours, to rattle the roof and break windows. I wouldn't be surprised if that were true.

During the term of Mr F. J. Gillen, my father's predecessor at Alice Springs, Mrs Gillen brought a white woman servant from Adelaide to help her. She wasn't very young and she was very deaf, but that didn't worry George—he became as smitten as a lovelorn youth and pursued her ardently. But his mighty voice could not register the dulcet tones of courting. He knew no sound softer than fortissimo, and his booming endearments were the joy of the station.

Eventually they were engaged and decided to be married in Adelaide. At Oodnadatta, on the trip south for the wedding, the lady didn't feel well. George suggested a little whisky, but a little led to a lot. She had so many "tastes" that night that she was still drunk when the train reached Adelaide. George saw her safely into the care of her family and said goodbye for ever. Later he discovered she had gone to Alice Springs, as far away as she could from regular supplies of whisky, to dry out from a prolonged period of alcoholism. When she got off the buggy at Oodnadatta she also went off the wagon.

That was the end of serious love affairs for George, although he retained a twinkle in his eyes. "No more women for me," he used to say. "A man might find himself hitched to a brewery."

Miss Easom also made an impression on Bob Crann, our other driver. I ought to have been too young to notice such things but perhaps I was a precocious child! In any case, I remember that we eventually reached Charlotte Waters telegraph station, the only one we would see before Alice Springs, and where we rested for a day or so, Bob Crann spent his entire time in the blacksmith's shop. When he emerged he presented to Miss Easom a crescent-shaped brooch which he had made from coins with the initials B.L.E. engraved neatly in the centre. This was his rough equivalent of a box of chocolates or a bottle of perfume and I'm sure Miss Easom was suitably impressed.

Charlotte Waters was one of a chain of telegraph stations spaced about two hundred miles apart all the way from Port Augusta to Darwin. Several of them, like Marree, Alice Springs, and Powell Creek, were "repeaters"—stations where the Morse signals passing constantly along the line were boosted in strength so that they might be received in Adelaide with sufficient volume to be understood. The officer-in-charge at Charlotte Waters was Patrick Byrne, who apparently did not share George Hablett's and Bob Crann's interest in a pretty girl. He welcomed us warmly enough but then spoilt it all by saying he'd have to move farther out—as if anywhere could be farther out than Charlotte Waters!

"Why?" he was asked.

"The place is becoming overrun by women," he replied tartly.

Charlotte Waters telegraph station was an impressive structure of natural stone, with big rooms and small windows designed to give maximum protection against possible attack by hostile aborigines. We were still not out of the gibber country. To me it seemed that we had arrived at the end of the world. The aspect was truly dismaying and my earlier fears about what I might find at Alice Springs were refreshed. I'm not surprised that Charlotte Waters, sitting almost squarely on the boundary of South Australia and the Northern Territory, was subsequently abandoned and the station moved to Finke, a few miles from Horseshoe Bend. However, we had passed out of South Australia and each days drive now represented an increasing percentage of the remaining distance.

As though we hadn't had enough travel already, we made a detour from Charlotte Waters to visit Mr and Mrs Alex Ross, their son Alex Junior, and daughter Ruby at Crown Point station, which Mr Ross managed. It wasn't more than a day's drive off our track—in each direction, of course—and that, as we were soon to learn, was the nearest thing we were likely to have to next-door neighbours. We had a delightful break of a day and a half with the Ross family. The visit, for mother especially, was a charming interlude, as Mrs Ross was able to give her many valuable womanly hints on how to manage in this unknown land. There were few who knew it better than she did; with her husband she had lived on several scattered stations throughout Central Australia.

The history of the Centre was dripping from her veins, for she was connected with the earliest pioneers. She had been Miss Fanny Wallis, an aunt of Frank and Albert Wallis who opened the first general store in Alice Springs, then known as Stuart, a few years before our arrival. Later, as Wallis Fogarty's, it was the store when Alice Springs was a thriving township. In the early 1960s it was bought by an airline company which wanted the block of land, and so the shop closed down. Today you buy tourist travel where Frank Wallis once sold flour by the ton and treacle by the four-gallon tin.

Mrs Ross had "acquired" more family history when she married. Her husband was a son of John Ross, acknowledged to be the first man after John McDouall Stuart to reach Central Australia. When the South Australian Government decided to build the O.T. Line the only information they had about the country was that supplied by McDouall Stuart following his explorations in 1860 and 1861, and his eventual crossing of the continent in 1862. The South Australian Postmaster-General, Mr (later Sir) Charles Todd, commissioned John Ross in 1870 to make a survey of the proposed route. He was to be paid £450 a year (a good salary in those days) but Todd instructed that the men he took with him, except a qualified surveyor, were to be paid not more than £1/1/- a week. The surveyor was a Mr Harvey; the three men were Alfred Giles, who subsequently became famous in his own right, T. Crispe, and W. Hearn. It was Ross who named the Todd River after his boss, and two beauty spots, Jessie and Emily Gaps, were named after his daughters.

John Ross was regarded as an admirable explorer. He was a highly competent bushman, and tough and resourceful in overcoming the problems he met in opening up the waterless spaces of the interior. There is little doubt that his work merits more recognition than it has been given. Though Stuart was a marvellously hardy man and a tenacious explorer, his contribution was to prove that the continent could be crossed with horses. That work ended in 1862. Thereafter it was Ross who showed the way to settlement.

Many years later, I visited Frank Wallis's sister, Mrs Roberts, in Hyde Park, Adelaide. Then aged eighty-six and the only remaining member of the family, she knew John Ross well, and proudly showed me a photograph of him. "He was a lovely man," she said.

But that wasn't all the history we found at Crown Point. Alex Ross himself, as a youth of eighteen, had been a member of Ernest Giles's 1875 expedition from Beltana, near Lake Torrens, across the northern fringe of the Nullarbor Plain to Perth. On that journey Ross, by following a flock of birds, found and named the beautiful Queen Victoria Spring in the heart of the Great Victoria Desert.

Now here we were at Crown Point with him—and I was too young to understand or appreciate the hardships he had suffered. I remember walking around the old stone homestead and thinking, "Pooh! What an old place! I wouldn't like to live here." Mrs Ross had done her best to brighten the house with huge jars of gumtips. She was plump, attractive, and happy. A few years earlier she had entertained Vice-Royalty when Lord Kintore, the South Australian Governor, visited the station. Later Alex Ross became Inspector of Water Supplies for the South Australian and Federal Governments in the Northern Territory. An official record of his life ends with this entry: "He suffered injury to his spine through being thrown from a camel, and this accident led to his death."
There was more to it than that—in fact it was an epic story of the bush, and the authority for it is Alex Ross himself.

A visiting pastoralist who wished to examine vacant land north-east of Alice Springs engaged Ross and an aboriginal to take him there. The white men each had riding camels, but the aboriginal was perched on top of a powerful bull-camel loaded with packs carrying water and food. Riding a camel isn't the easiest mode of travel, especially without the support of a proper saddle, and it wasn't long before Ross noticed that the native had developed serious abrasions.

Ross pointed this out to the visitor, and asked that the native should be allowed to ride behind him in a double saddle on his camel. This idea was indignantly rejected. So Alex Ross, with typical kindness, gave the injured man his own camel and mounted the pack-carrier himself, leaving the double-saddle with one vacant seat.

As usual, the camels were linked with noselines and the trek resumed with the aboriginal leading. On the second day the noseline on the pack-camel became entangled in a mulga branch and broke. The big beast was frightened, bucked violently, and threw Ross many feet into the air. He fell heavily on his back but was able to remount and ride to the end of that day's stage.

Next morning Ross was very ill and knew that he was not fit to ride to Alice Springs, still two days away. So he sent the others ahead and rode alone to the near-by camp of a dogger whose horse-bells he had heard. This man took a message to another pioneer, Alf Turner, whose camp was twelve miles away, while Ross spread his blankets and waited for help. Turner answered the call immediately and when he arrived found Ross almost helpless on his blankets.

Turner, shocked at his condition, gave what first aid he could, prepared food and tea, and after making Ross as comfortable as possible rode all night to Bond Springs station. Soon after noon next day he was back with a vehicle which would carry the injured man to Alice Springs. On the way they rescued a well-sinker, Bob Plew, who had fallen forty feet to the bottom of a hole and fractured his back when he stepped into an unattended windlass bucket. Alf Turner climbed down the timbering of the well, strapped Plew to the bucket, then climbed hand over hand to the surface. He brought him to the top, put him in his own buckboard, and for the second time travelled all night to help an injured man. They reached the Australian Inland Mission hostel at Alice Springs next morning. Plew was cared for there and later sent to Adelaide, but he lived only long enough to reach hospital. Alex Ross only partly recovered and was never able to work again. He died less than two years later in the Home for Incurables in Adelaide.

That was still very much in the future on that cold May day when we were with the Ross family at Crown Point and, of course, none of us had any conception that Alex Ross would suffer such a violent and painful death. Our stay with them was a happy one, although my chief interest came from the discovery on their bookshelves of the entire "Elsie" series, the current romantic stories for girls. I read my way through them as quickly as possible and was still reading, oblivious of everything else, when I was forcibly thrust into the buggy to resume the drive to Alice Springs.

On and on we went, the horses as weary as we, especially when they had to pull their heavy loads through the dreaded Depot Sandhills. At least we were out of the flat gibber country. The sandhills were interspersed with red country where mulga and desert oaks, spinifex and often good grazing land relieved the tedium. On we went and on, the sand still crawling up the buggy wheels, the traces and the chains creaking and rattling as they had when we left Oodnadatta more than a week ago. The horses' ribs were beginning to show; they were feeling the strain of the trip, but George Hablett assured us all that they would still be pulling when we reached Alice Springs where they would soon recover their condition for future journeys.

On and on, across the Finke, a broad sweep of dry sand which would become a torrent in the rainy season—or so I was assured, for I found it difficult to believe that enough rain ever fell in this country to make creeks and rivers flow. On we went past Horseshoe Bend, a broad sweep in the river which has retained that name on today's maps, and through more seemingly endless sandhills. They were in serried ranks, some fifty feet high, all starkly red and caressed by the south-east trade winds which caused "wavelets" to form on their smooth slopes. Fortunately many of the sandhills ran in the same direction as ours and we were able to drive along deep valleys. Nevertheless, it seemed that we were frequently crossing others. My eyes were sore from looking at sand, but I knew the trip was in its last stages and I tried not to complain. In any case, I might have been ashamed to do so, for my younger brothers and sister had travelled marvellously well, and my mother must have been under constant strain while caring for a baby and other small children during a fortnight's buggy ride.

On and on, the horses now walking more often than they trotted, their heads low, their animal alertness gone. One midday we came to a cattle station known as Alice Well, run by William Hayes and his family, and we were invited for lunch—but if I expected something more than salt beef and bread I was disappointed. An impression remains of several tall, tanned young men and their two sisters, all of them helping their parents to carve a station from the wilderness. They were among the first of the Inland pioneers. Most of the children had been born there and knew all there was to know of bushcraft. Undoolya station, which they bought later, still belongs to the Hayes family, and today is managed by Ted Hayes junior, a grandson of William Hayes, one of the original settlers.

My most vivid memory of Alice Well is that the dining room walls were papered entirely with the picture sections of weekly newspapers, a wonderful idea which kept me entranced throughout the meal. Fancy being able to read a wall, I thought!

Subsequently I heard about two men who reached the Hayes' home on a cold and wet night. All members of the family, including Mrs Hayes and the girls, were away in mustering camps, but an aboriginal who was there invited the men to camp for the night in the warm house, assuring them that Mr and Mrs Hayes would wish it. Grateful for the shelter, they had settled down to sleep when they were awakened by the barking of dogs. The family had returned unexpectedly for a dry night's rest. The interlopers explained how they came to be in possession and offered to move out but the Hayes laughed at the idea. They insisted upon remaining in the open and cheerfully spread their camping gear. I wonder how much of that kind of bush hospitality remains today?

And so, at last, after nearly three weeks, the great day came when we would arrive at Alice Springs.

The MacDonnell Ranges had been in view for several days, looming gradually closer and bigger, but losing little of their colours which changed so quickly with the direction of the sun's rays. It was during these last two or three days that we all began using again a word which had slipped from our vocabularies since leaving the Flinders Ranges outside Port Augusta. That word was "beautiful." For a full fortnight there had been nothing in the landscape to suggest anything but ugliness; but now, suddenly, my mother exclaimed, "Oh, isn't that beautiful!" And we all knew that, though we hadn't expressed it, the beauty of the dormant heart of the continent had impressed itself upon us, too.

"You really haven't seen much of it yet," my father said. "Here you will find a wonderland of chasms and gorges and valleys that are as dramatic as anything I have seen. I wouldn't be surprised if, one day, this becomes a great tourist centre."

Sixty years later it had become just that, with thousands of people flocking there, some from the other side of the world.

As we drove over open country before entering Heavitree Gap and passing along the bed of the Todd River, groups of kangaroos appeared as though they had come out to welcome us. Not many had yet been killed and so they seemed quite tame. A number of big greys and reds faced each other in mock combat, delighting us with boxing attitudes that were almost human.

"They look like men moving through the trees," my mother said. "And look at those fighting—this could be a great tournament!"

We passed through Heavitree Gap, not more than a hundred yards wide, and into the centre of the MacDonnell Ranges. On our left was Mount Gillen, named for his father by the man who was my father's predecessor for nine years.

Ahead of us was the winding Todd River, liberally overgrown with ghost gums and river gums, the biggest trees we had seen for three weeks; beyond that was a plain stretching north for several miles to the next tiers of the MacDonnells, and in the middle distance was the small township we had waited so long and driven so far to see. We were all highly excited and, risking paternal displeasure, I stood up in the buggy and pointed.

"There's Alice Springs!" I shouted. "I can see it!" And then turning to my father, I said, "Thanks for bringing me. It looks beautiful."

Chapter Three

ALICE...WE GET TO KNOW HER

THE ALICE WAS STILL IN HER TWENTIES. EVEN so she was a lovely young woman in 1899 and already showing promise of the elegant maturity she would one day reach. Her hair was done with a garland of wild flowers and ghost gums. Namatjira purple, invented by the sun some years before the artist, was thickly applied to the surrounding hills. But there were times when Alice seemed rather faded. Midday in summer was a trying time when all the colour drained from her face. Dust storms came occasionally and hid her beneath a layer of fine red powder that was most unbecoming. Despite these vicissitudes, these seasonal moments when she wasn't quite herself, Alice's tranquil charm converted all of us to her side. Her very comeliness made us soon forget the deep scars engraved on our souls by the soulless desert we had crossed. Before long we were happy to be with her, to discover and share her joys, and to have her keep us. In the months and years that followed, as my diary reminds me, I rode out almost daily to find the hidden facets of her character. This quest was never forced upon me, but was something I liked to do. The only time I felt any unease—that unhappy feeling of being away from home—was the one occasion when we set out for a holiday in Adelaide—not because I did not enjoy the change, but because it meant a dual crossing by buggy of the awful sand-and-gibber land.

In my time the township was known as Stuart, and I rather regret that the name was changed. I've been told that this happened when the old post office at the Alice Springs telegraph station, two miles away, was eventually transferred to the growing village. The postmaster continued to use the Alice Springs postmark to frank all mail and the name was also used as the originating office for telegrams. This usage became so common that eventually the name Stuart was forgotten. The town that is Alice was on its way to modest fame. For this reason, and for the sake of clarity, I shall henceforth refer to Alice Springs only, while hoping that its given name will never be forgotten.

The villagers, at that time, were few indeed—perhaps not more than twelve or thirteen. As we passed through the village on our arrival we first saw Mounted Constable Charles Brookes, his wife, and four children at the Police Camp on the southern side of Heavitree Gap. He must have been one of the loneliest policemen in the world, especially as his duties frequently required him to be long distances away from home on horse and camel patrols. Some of my most vivid recollections are of Constable Brookes returning to Alice Springs with lines of aboriginal prisoners chained by the neck. They never failed to stir in my youthfully democratic breast a deep sense of outrage and revulsion. Nor did I like it any more because each time I was reminded of the horror I had seen at Oodnadatta. When I protested to the adults, in my childish way, that what we were seeing was inhumane, I was told that

Arriving back from leave in 1905. Harry Kunoth driving, mother beside him nursing Edna

Alice Springs' first tennis court, near the Stuart Arms Hotel

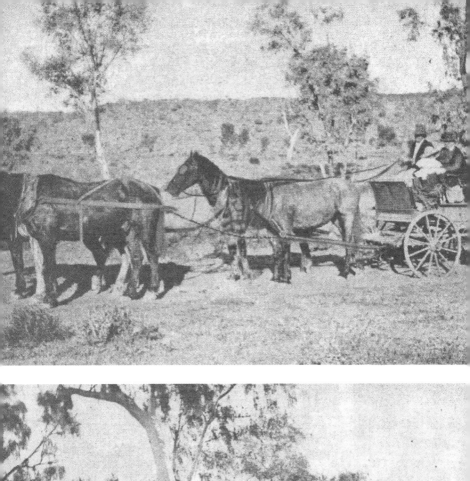

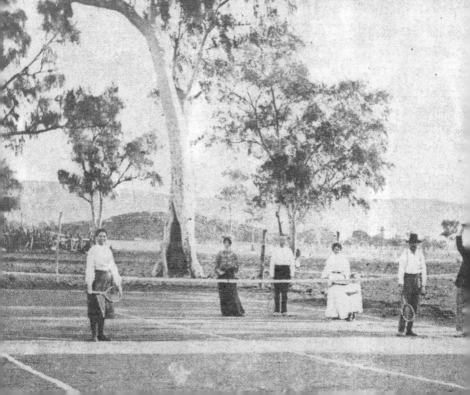

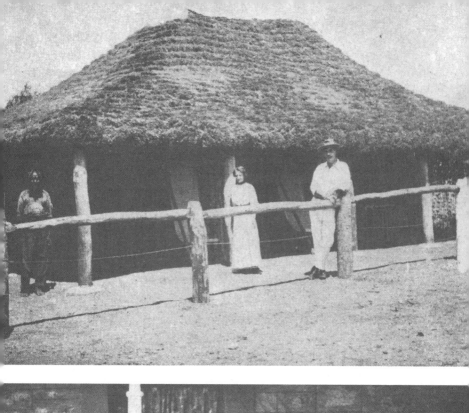

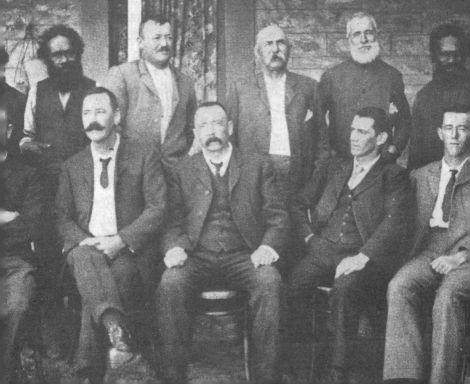

nothing could be done about it—the prisoners and witnesses would run away while being brought in if they weren't secured. The practice of chaining men was abolished in the Northern Territory only a few years ago, so we are told. But I wouldn't be surprised if they are sometimes still chained in the name of the law in remote areas where the law is not likely to see. In case it should ever be forgotten that human beings were treated in this way, I have preserved photographs of chained men. I have also a photograph of a log cabin—a shack with but a single entrance and no other ventilation—which stood beside the infant police station. This, to Her Majesty's discredit, was Her Majesty's Alice Springs gaol—and I'm sure that Queen Victoria would not have been amused had she known of its existence.

Only one white woman lived in the township itself. She was Mrs Charles Meyers, whose husband had established a saddlery business. These days new townships spring up around roadhouses and service stations. The villages of 1899 could manage without them, even without a butcher or a baker, but few could do without a saddler. These shops had a distinctive aroma of tanned leather, resin, and twine that has disappeared from the catalogue of smells one encounters each day. The pastrycook's shop, the delicatessen, the pharmacy, the drapery, the grocery, all give off smells that almost any modern housewife can recognize instantly. But I wonder how many would know where they were if pushed into a darkened saddlery.

We did not meet Mrs Meyers until a few weeks later. She was eighty miles away at Hermannsburg Lutheran mission station

My uncle and aunt, Mr and Mrs Ernest Allchurch, and staff, at their cottage, built on the telegraph station in 1905

The O.T. Line staff at Alice Springs. At rear: Harry Kunoth (against post), Jim Rodda, Billy Crick. Front: Bill Perry, Ern Allchurch, T. A. Bradshaw, Charles Lamshed, Leslie Spicer

for the birth of her second child, Herman John. Women were there to help her, the wives of intrepid missionaries who had been in the district for more than twenty years. Otherwise, Mrs Brookes would have had to cope single-handed, and she had four of her own to care for. I was too young to understand the fear these women must have known upon the approach of each confinement, well aware that if the birth should be complicated the nearest doctor was ten days' travel away at Oodnadatta or Marree. My own mother gave birth to three more children while we were at Alice Springs, attended only by Mrs Meyers. Not that there was much difference when her eighth child was born, back in Adelaide, before a doctor reached her!

The Stuart Arms, now an ornate five-star hotel, was then a modest structure of stone and iron, about the size of an average house, with a post and rail hitching-fence around the veranda. Buggies and wagons parked outside in what is now Todd Street. It was then a forest of gums. I remember Mr Gunther, the publican, who looked just as a publican should—a portly, florid man with a scarlet cummerbund swathed around his middle. He waved politely as we passed. Soon the hotel was bought by Charlie South, who married and brought his wife there. She and my mother were firm friends.

Standing beside Mr Gunther was George Wilkinson, who managed Wallis's store on the opposite corner. This was also a stone building with an iron roof and a veranda supported by bush posts. It had a stone chimney, the inevitable hitching-rail, and a sign on the roof which announced: WALLIS'S STORE. AGENCY AND DEPOT.

Fred Raggatt's store was also near the hotel, but he was nowhere to be seen. A short distance from Wallis's store there were two houses, one empty and the other occupied by George Wilkinson.

That was Stuart. One hotel, two stores, three houses...and nothing more until we reached our own home, the telegraph station, two miles distant. A tiny village, true enough, but all the building materials except the stone had been carried more than three hundred miles on the backs of camels. The roads were bush tracks sparkling with mica. The villagers obtained water from wells, although the Bradshaw family, bits of snobs, had the misnamed waterhole—Alice Springs—which wasn't a spring at all.

Our horse-and-buggy cavalcade passed out of the township almost as soon as we'd entered it. The only noise we heard was that to which we had been accustomed for the past fortnight—the draw and creak of traces and chains and the clank of iron tyres on the micaceous ground. Our two vehicles, the buggy and the buckboard, represented the entire "stream" of traffic. When our dust settled behind us we could see that the village was barren of movement and, it seemed, almost of life. Gunther and Wilkinson, standing at the hotel door; had acknowledged us but now dropped back into a torpid somnolence apparently encouraged by the warm sun. I suppose our arrival was the biggest event in Alice Springs for some months, perhaps for years, and yet it caused only a minor ripple of excitement. I felt that we should have been greeted by bunting, a welcoming committee, and an escort of outriders to accompany us along the valley of the Todd; after all, it isn't every day that the arrival of one family increases a town's population by fifty per cent.

We crossed the Todd, drove through a pleasant spot along the banks known as Middle Park, and followed the winding river as it entered the sandy stone country of the MacDonnells. And there, perched on high ground above the spring in the river bed, was the telegraph station, our home for the next nine and a half years, and the end of a long, long buggy ride.

Both my mother and Miss Easom were quite as excited as I was. For them, the trip had been a constant strain. I had been able to relax and do as I pleased in often vain attempts to relieve the tedium, but they had nursed the younger children and had always been on the alert to ensure that no one fell overboard. Now they laughed gaily and patted and embraced each other—the tension eased and their spirits fully restored.

They waved to the big group of aborigines in their camp on the bank of the river. Dozens of dogs welcomed us with a cacophony of yelping. The entire community came to life: the dogs from their one-eyed sleep in the shade, the elders from their segregated "court" near the centre of the camp, and piccaninnies of all sizes emerged with mothers, aunts, sisters, brothers, and cousins, scrambling on all fours from bark wurlies to stare at us shyly and wave diffidently. The black boys we saw that day are now elders in the Aranda tribe, with a certain education and sophistication, but I thought of them as the most primitive children on earth. They were dirty in the extreme, and I was shocked to see that many were quite naked—a state to be altered at once on my father's instruction but by my mother's work. There must have been a hundred and fifty natives in the camp, and a third of them had no clothes at all. One of my mother's first duties was to make sixty serge skirts on a hand-operated sewing machine she had brought with her.

Before dismounting we were greeted with a wave by a little old white man named Billy Crick, the station gardener, who was busy attending to his vegetables. We had passed a stockyard where twenty or thirty horses crowded to the rail to greet their kind and perhaps to inspire them to a final effort, for the tired teams really did bring us up with a flourish in front of the station buildings. These were made of stone and were the most substantial of any kind that we had seen since leaving Port Augusta.

I must say that I was suitably impressed by the obvious importance of the telegraph station. It consisted of nine main stone buildings, with two or three smaller ones, all huddled together in a compact group and representing a bigger community than the village itself. My youthful pride was inflated; it was an honour to be there and to be able to say, when asked, that one lived at the Telegraph Station—with capital letters, if you please.

Apart from my father, who was officer-in-charge, there were four other operators: Jim Field, Phillip Squire, Mr Middleton, and Mr Jago. They came out to welcome us, and Jim Field, the senior, showed mother our quarters; if a little rough and ready, they were at least substantial and are now preserved as a national museum by the Northern Territory Reserves Board. He also introduced the two aboriginal women who had worked for Mrs Gillen and were to be among our inheritances. Someone with a classical imagination had named one of them Tryphena, and that has been perpetuated in Tryphena Gorge, now a popular tourist attraction. Mother was given much advice on how to manage the native women, emphasis being laid on the trouble she would have if she "spoilt" them, that is, treated them with unaccustomed kindness. However, the turnover in these primitive domestics was quite high and, of course, their temperaments varied. Mother found that she could not treat one as she could another, that some responded better to firmness than to kindness, and that others were so dull they were quite impossible. But there was plenty of time for my mother to learn; she was doing very well when we left almost a decade later, having by then "adopted," dressed, treated, and nursed dozens of them.

So there we were—a small self-contained community of telegraphists and linemen, a stockman, a governess, our family, and the man who was perhaps the most important of all, a professional cook named Alfred Lloyd. He had to cope with distance and lack of supplies—and a complete absence of variety—yet keep the staff happy by giving them adequate, if not appetizing, food. I did not envy him his job.

The native staff included a rather elastic number of horseboys, shepherds for cows and sheep, hewers of wood and carriers of water, scullerymaids for the staff kitchen, and two housemaids and a nursegirl in our home. I'm not too sure what the nursegirl's duties were, for mother wasn't keen on letting her too near the younger children. But the housemaids, Dolly and Tryph, were reasonably efficient.

At that time none of the natives understood the value of money, a failing which was to embarrass their future eminent tribesman Albert Namatjira, who was chronically bankrupt even when earning up to £7,000 a year. So they worked for their food and a stick of dark tobacco a day. The government also supplied shirts and trousers for the men employed on the station, but these were often gambled or given away to people not entitled to them.

Our quarters consisted of three large living and sleeping rooms surrounded by a wide veranda which helped deflect the direct rays of the summer sun but did little to reduce a temperature frequently above one hundred and ten degrees. A kitchen and small dining room were detached from the living rooms to minimize heat from the wood stove. Even so, the atmosphere was often so stifling that some artificial means of cooling, or at least stirring a breeze, had to be used. Electricity was then still a thing of the future, especially in Alice Springs, so we improvised with an intriguing punkah—the first I had ever seen. It was made from narrow boards, frilled calico, and ropes which passed through holes in the wall. An aboriginal was stationed outside to pull slowly and regularly on the rope—and, lo, we had a primitive fan. The punkah-wallah, however, was inclined to let us down on the hottest days when he was most needed; the heat and the regular motion apparently had a soporific effect and the punkah would gradually slow down until it stopped altogether. Our mealtimes were frequently punctuated with orders to this unseen black man that he should wake up and do his job. He'd resume half heartedly, but it was no use—once sleep got the better of him he was never fully conscious again and in due course we learnt to save our breath.

The punkah was supposed to have the secondary effect of keeping the flies at bay. Anyone who has been to Central Australia will know that when I say flies I mean clouds of flies—countless millions of them. They were the bane of our existence, especially during meals, and we had no deathdealing insecticide sprays. By creating a breeze the punkah did reduce this nuisance; so when the gentleman in charge went to sleep we had two reasons for being annoyed.

One day a portly matron named Polly, aware of the problem, offered her services as fly-swisher-in-chief during meals. She demonstrated her technique with a leafy bough and pressed her claim for the job by saying, "All-day me bin shepherd'em flies longa Mitta Gillen." But father declined with thanks. Apparently he preferred to take his chances with the flies rather than risk having his food flicked away by a switch. Later we transferred our eating quarters to one of the larger rooms and before a meal the entire family was marshalled to "shepherd'em flies" in the general direction of the window. Wire screens were unknown. If father had asked for them he'd probably have been told they were an unnecessary luxury; in any case, they would have taken valuable loading space on the camel trains required for more vitally needed supplies.

For several days we had fun exploring the station and its wonderful works, and we made some exciting discoveries. I remember that one of these gave me the kind of thrill that today's Hollywood publicity men would call "spine-chilling," but it didn't last long and I can't recall any sense of insecurity or impending doom. We found within a few minutes of our arrival that our rooms were fitted with loopholes. These could have been passed off as miniature windows if anyone was sensitive about childish fears. However, it was thought better to tell us exactly what they were for, if only to induce in us a proper respect for danger. The loopholes were firing positions for rifles which it had been intended should be aimed at hostile aborigines. Our bedrooms, in fact, were miniature forts designed to let loose invisible death if ever we were attacked by the natives. For the same reason the operators' quarters were built around a quadrangular courtyard equipped with gates which were supposed to afford the staff complete safety from spears and other weapons.

The expense of building all the telegraph stations in this fashion had not been undertaken without good reason. Tragic proof of the hostility of the natives was seen at Barrow Creek, our nearest neighbour, on 22nd February, 1874, only twenty-five years before our arrival. At eight o'clock that night the officer-in-charge, Mr J. L. Stapleton, was sitting outside the station with five members of his staff and a policeman, Mounted Constable Gason. The heat was intense and they had gone out for some fresh air to the south-west side of the building, farthest from the iron gate at the rear, and also farthest from the flat-top hills behind the station where aborigines could remain hidden until dark and then move stealthily down without being seen.

Suddenly the white men were surprised by a volley of spears. They dashed for the safety of their courtyard, but as they reached the gateway a lineman named Franks was speared in the back, the weapon entering his heart. He staggered into the kitchen where he collapsed and died immediately. Stapleton got six feet inside the gate before receiving four spear wounds from which he died next day. His assistant, Ernest Flint, and the policeman, Sam Gason, were both wounded; but with others they got inside the building and poured a volley of shots through the loopholes—identical with those in our rooms—to clear the field. Flint, though wounded, then went to the Morse key and sent word of the attack to Alice Springs from where it was flashed to Adelaide. On hearing of the tragedy, Charles Todd sent his carriage for Stapleton's wife, who was living in North Adelaide. Doctor Gosse was called to the G.P.O. and gave instructions for treatment which were relayed to Barrow

Creek. But from the start it had been obvious that Stapleton was doomed, and he was aware of it himself. Against the wishes of his friends, he insisted on being lifted to the Morse key; as his strength ebbed he tapped out a last message to his wife which, Todd translated for her:

"God bless you and the children."

His hand fell from the key and in a short while he was dead.

There is a grim sequel to this story. A punitive party of police and white bushmen was sent out to avenge the dead men. They ranged over thousands of square miles of country then inhabited only by aborigines and shot every one they found—men, women, and children. One of the peaks in the Harts Range, away to the east of Barrow Creek, is named Blackfellows' Bones, and a watercourse near by is named Skull Creek, both names a reminder of this massacre. Flint was later officer-in-charge of Alice Springs station, preceding Skinner and later Gillen, and he died there. His was the first grave in the little station cemetery. I saw it there—and years later, at the home of the late Alex Ross, I saw the telegram he sent telling of the attack upon the Barrow Creek station. It is now preserved in the South Australian Archives.

But as we lay in bed at night with the south-east trade winds blowing through the loopholes I was not concerned that similar attacks might be made on us. The Alice Springs station had never been attacked by the Aranda. They were close neighbours of the Kaiditj at Barrow Creek but were less belligerent. The Kaiditj perhaps acquired their hostility from the warlike Warramunga, their northern neighbours, who barred McDouall Stuart's way at Attack Creek in 1861 and paid the price with the lives of tribesmen. Rather than being afraid of them, I always regarded the Aranda as friends. They were extremely primitive and dirty and we were forbidden to play with them, but in the manner of children everywhere we found ways around that rule when those in authority weren't watching. In any event, I was never troubled by the slightest fear that one day my family and I might be massacred while we slept.

One of the other fascinating aspects of the station was that in the staff kitchen Cookie Lloyd kept a blanket-lined box in which slept a two-year-old part-aboriginal girl. Her mother had died when she was born. As the child of a mixed-race union she was unwanted by the tribes people. They left her to die in the bush and attempted to hasten the process by filling her mouth and nose with sand. But Cookie Lloyd rescued her and installed her in his big warm kitchen. There she lived and grew like a carefree young puppy. Father said repeatedly that she must go to the camp to live with the aboriginal women; but as none of them were prepared to look after her my father always relented and allowed her to stay with Cookie. There, like Topsy, she grew into a wild and defiant creature. She wore a few cast-off rags and, towards her master at least, behaved like a pet dog. But otherwise she was always in mischief of some kind and frequent inquests were held into her misdemeanours. At one time the nanny goats we kept as a stand in for the cows were mysteriously short of milk. My brothers, Jack and Mort, then a little older, hid near the sheep pen one day and unravelled the mystery—our tame young vixen was getting to the goats before the lubras whose job it was to milk them. They caught her redhanded with a jam tin full of milk and gave chase. As they were about to grab her flapping rags she turned and threw the milk in their faces. While the boys wiped it out of their eyes she escaped into the hills like a young wallaby. I'm sure Mort and Jack thought it worthwhile fun.

We called her Mumpaguila. Fifty years later my sister Consie and I visited her in the Royal Adelaide Hospital where she lay dying of cancer in the throat. Gone was the utterly wild girl of the bush; in her place we found a dignified, patient woman who had married and raised her own family. She had been flown to Adelaide in three hours over country through which we toiled for nearly three weeks.

In his tall white cap and big white apron Cookie Lloyd looked like a professional chef, but I'm afraid that was the most professional part of him. He made quite good bread and yeast buns—a dozen were sent over to us almost every day—but he was a dismal failure at preparing everyday menus for young men with ravenous appetites. The word "variety" just wasn't part of his vocabulary. Food, in his view, was something eaten to keep people alive. Cooking was therefore a necessary trade. But he had never learnt that good cooks could convert the commonest ingredients into palatable dishes varied by disguise. His meat was boiled or baked, his vegetables were ungarnished, and his desserts—what he called "puddin'—had to be eaten to be believed. For six days in every week the poor men got sago, made with water and nothing else, and known sardonically to them as "slide." I suppose that was because it wobbled like a jelly and, unless one was careful, it went for a slide off the plate and on to the table. The window of the staff dining room faced ours across the yard. Cookie Lloyd's confections must have been the subject of conversation between us, because we often watched a silent pantomime which had us in hysterics. The dining room window would fly open and a dish of slide be held aloft. "Here it is again," was the message. The man holding the dish would look at it despairingly for a moment, then disappear. On one occasion, to our great delight, the despair flared into rebellion and the offending dish of slide was thrown into the yard.

One of the men was once given two eggs, a tremendous treat in a country where fowls were almost as scarce as fish. Rather than eat them for breakfast, he thought he'd share them by asking Cookie Lloyd to make a milk pudding. At the appropriate moment the pudding was produced—good old slide with the two eggs nestling neatly on top. Even so, Cookie apparently wasn't as bad as one cook we heard of. When the station manager he cooked for complained of the sameness of the menu he said, "Well, I was going to give you blancmange for a change today, but there wasn't any dripping."

Our own food, which mother cooked, was prepared from the same basic ingredients as the staff's, and although there was sometimes an understandable lack of variety it was generally palatable and enjoyable. Meat was served three times a day—chops, steaks, and roasts, and occasionally a Burdekin Duck for breakfast. This was a favourite bush meal (sometimes also known as Kimberley Oysters): slices of cold roast or corned beef were dipped in a batter of flour, baking powder, milk, and chopped onions. They were then fried in hot fat. The result—golden brown fritters.

We seldom saw fresh fruit. The varieties that could survive a camel trip from Oodnadatta were few. Tinned fruit was plentiful during the first part of our ration year, but towards the end it was sometimes absent from our menus. Flour, tea, sugar, tinned goods, medical supplies, blankets, and clothing—everything needed for the maintenance of the station—came on camels only once a year.

Mother and father spent days preparing our order many months before they could hope to receive it. It was sent on the mail coach to Adelaide merchants who bought on our behalf any goods they couldn't supply from stock, packed it all in large wooden cases, and consigned it by the first camel. Considering the weeks they were on the track, and that each crate had to be unloaded every night and hoisted on to the camel's back again next morning, it was a remarkable tribute to the firm that nothing was ever broken.

I can remember mother and father making inventories of everything in the house, and then stock-taking before each order was due to be placed. Maybe bales of striped galatea and finer material were needed for boys' blouses and girls' dresses. Perhaps cups and saucers had been broken during the year and had to be replaced. They may have wanted clothing or a few luxuries for us that couldn't be obtained locally. But they had to be extremely careful in such matters because if we exceeded our "free" allowance, camel freight was more expensive than air freight today. A pound of cheese could cost as much as £1 to land in Alice Springs.

The shopping list, written on many sheets of paper, seemed endless. And the quantities were enormous, especially of such basic commodities as flour and sugar. I imagine that the station staff and the aborigines required hundreds, perhaps thousands, of pounds of flour to keep us going through the year.

No besieged legion getting its first glimpse of relief troops shouted more enthusiastically than we did on the day our annual stores arrived. Everyone stopped work. We deserted the schoolroom and our governess, who was just as excited; aborigines came running from the creek; the staff stood around while my father ceremoniously took delivery of the station's goods. Slowly, silently, the great packing cases creaking as they swayed, the long string of camels came padding into the station compound, looking haughty and slightly disdainful. Each was linked to the other by a cord attached to a nosepeg. The Afghan driver went to each in turn and pulled on the cord.

"Hooshta! Hooshta!" he cried.

Protestingly at first, and yet with a great willingness to be relieved of their burdens, the animals knelt, grunting and sometimes squealing, then folded their hind legs and squatted on the ground. The great packs, weighing as much as five hundred pounds, were unlashed—and then these marvellous beasts of burden could rest for a few days.

I have no idea what we and the whole of the Inland would have done without camels. They were stand-offish, unlovable, smelly in the extreme—and yet indispensable. Professor Baldwin Spencer, in *Across Australia,* says he travelled two thousand miles on camels but parted from them without the slightest regret. Perhaps that wasn't altogether the camels' fault: during his first expedition he did not realize the tremendous difference between a pack camel and a riding camel—a difference as great, I've been told, as between a draught horse and a hack. He had ridden a pack camel all the way.

Some men grew attached to them. I remember the government geologist and surveyor H. Y. L. Brown, arriving at the station on a beautiful white riding camel named Jessie Darling. She was such an attractive animal that he persuaded mother and our governess to take a ride. He had his drawing board fixed in front of the saddle so that he could work without dismounting.

Alex Ross also thought highly of his camels; this, I discovered later, was common to anyone who understood their worth in the grim outback. I'm sure that no other animal could have carried the loads they did through such gruelling conditions. Elephants, perhaps? Could they have crossed the desert from Oodnadatta to Alice Springs, on time-table frequency, and remained tractable and manageable? I doubt it; they belong in the big river country and the steaming jungles.

I can't say that I was fond of camels. They were ugly and smelly and I thought they could be treacherous. Our horses didn't like them either, presumably because they gave off the wild-beast smell that terrifies domestic animals. I was often surprised when riding one of my horses to find that it suddenly jibbed, sniffed the air, and tried to turn back. Invariably, when that happened, we would meet a string of camels farther on, sometimes a long way from the point where the scent was first noticeable to the horse.

Still, we certainly welcomed the string bringing our yearly supplies. All hands got to work at once, opening cases and carrying goods to storerooms. We'd almost topple into the cases head first in our eagerness. Even such mundane things as groceries were a thrill when they came only once a year.

One of our delights was to visit old Billy Crick in his vegetable garden on the bank of the river. As a producer of vegetables the garden had many peers. The soil was poor and was made poorer by pepper trees surrounding the garden. Billy Crick was a kindly old man—small, gnarled, weatherbeaten—and he lived alone in a hut under the trees. We liked talking to him because he was a member of the opposition and could be relied upon never to agree with any simple statement.

If I said, "The cabbages look well Billy," he could be guaranteed to reply, "Well, I dunno, they don't make no 'ears. I putt'en in three months ago, and look at 'em!"

But if I said, "Those carrots haven't come on too well Billy," he would say, "I putt'en in only six weeks ago. They're doin' fine."

Billy and the moon were on the most intimate of terms. He knew just what the weather would be from the way "she come in," that is, on its back or right side up, though once he admitted that he didn't like the way "she was carryin' on" at all. I must say that Billy was generally right with his weather forecasts—but weren't we all? Any eight-year old child could predict it almost with certainty. Seven-eighths of every year was fine, and we knew that blue skies meant fine days. When clouds began to build up it was an even-money bet that rain would develop. Even if it didn't, we had a fair chance of being right most of the time.

These three elderly men—Billy Crick, Cookie Lloyd, and George Hablett the stockman and handyman—were extremely patient and kind with us, as most bushmen are with children. George was our favourite, and we loved visiting him in the men's hut. He had decorated it with a frieze of coloured illustrations from a fashion journal—lovely ladies with impossible waists and huge leg-of-mutton sleeves. We could never understand why he had gone to the trouble of pasting them around the wall, for they gave him no pleasure. On the contrary, they infuriated him. He'd sit on his bunk, scornfully pointing his pipe at one or the other: "Now just take a look at her. A sack of flour tied in the middle, that's what she is! And look at her!... and her!...enough to make a man spit!" Or was it all a pose? Did he hanker, perhaps, for the bright lights and the cities of fashionable women? One never really knew...

I wouldn't like anyone to think that young children living in Alice Springs at the turn of the century were condemned to boredom or underprivileged in the matter of fun. There were simple joys around us that often made me feel I wouldn't want to change places with a princess. We had to look for our fun, but it wasn't hard to find. One of my greatest delights, as a girl of eight, was to help George Hablett in the blacksmith's shop on a cold day. Working the huge bellows up and down; making the fire glow in the forge; watching the horseshoes gradually turning red, then white-hot; standing wide-eyed and completely fascinated as George seized them in great tongs and plunged them into a wooden trough of water, where they hissed and gave off clouds of steam; then to watch carefully as he hammered a shoe into shape to fit a horse standing patiently in the roofed yard outside. This was absorbing fun that the average child could not share. And to see George actually shoeing a horse...what a treat that was! He rasped their hoofs almost as tenderly as if giving a pedicure and fitted the shoe until it sat snugly, then quickly hammered a few nails into the hoof to hold the shoe in place. That horrified me at first. I was sure the horse must feel those nails being driven into its foot but I was reassured.

"Don't be silly," one of the men told me. "Old George wouldn't ill-treat a horse any more than he would a child. And he's never been known to swear at a cow, which is even more remarkable."

The strongest threat George could make to a restive horse was to roar in its ear with his booming voice: "By golly, if you're not quiet I'll swaller yer!" One, a semi-draught, must have thought he was going to. George gave its leg such a mighty heave that the astonished animal landed on its back. If that seems far-fetched it should be said that he was an immensely strong man. He was known to have lifted a six-hundred-pound packing case from a wagon to the ground and to have let it down so gently that it scarcely stirred the dust.

I loved to watch him making spokes and buggy wheels and fitting the iron tyre which he also made in the smithy. This was highly skilled work, yet in those days it wasn't thought unusual. We also had fun watching him pave the verandas with stone from the near-by hills. To cart it from a heap George used a small cart drawn by a draught horse on long traces. But he acted as "shafter" himself; he actually got in between the shafts, lifted them, and did his share of pulling. In fact, most people believed that George did more work than the horse. Certainly he was always working, as might be imagined of someone who had seventy horses and three hundred cattle on his hands. The horses were used primarily for taking maintenance gangs and material to places needing repair along the O.T. Line. The cattle were purely for our own meat supply. There was also a herd of two hundred sheep. A bullock was slaughtered once a week in winter and a sheep a day in summer when the cattle were too poor. Occasionally a goat was killed, too. This mutton was intended for the aborigines, but if it was young enough Cookie Lloyd often slipped some of it into our rations believing we'd be none the wiser.

The only rickety thing about George Hablett was his English. Schoolboy howlers were to be expected from him almost daily, but "expected" was one word he didn't know. On an occasion when the Todd River flooded suddenly George said he hadn't "digested" it. He was always "insulting" people—his version of "consulting." I think he was quite incapable of insulting anyone or anything, with the possible exception of threatening to "swaller" a horse, and we came to love him as a very dear friend. He was certainly one of the chief contributors to our diversions and, as such, has remained strongly in my memory for more than sixty years.

Chapter Four

WALKABOUTS AND TALKABOUTS

THE FIRST DAYS AND WEEKS OF OUR STAY PASSED slowly. If I'd known then that we were to be in Alice Springs for more than nine years I'm sure I'd have been very depressed. But by the time the months had stretched into the first year we had settled down with plenty to keep us occupied and entertained.

Primarily, there were school lessons for me, and, before long, for the younger members of the family too. Nowadays parents hesitate before taking children to smaller towns and districts that are not well served by schools. Thousands leave the country every year for big cities which supposedly offer better academic opportunities. But my parents seemed unconcerned that I was being taken to a place that would be hundreds of miles from the nearest schoolhouse; they simply took a governess along and hoped that, for a few shillings a week, she might be able to impart some of her own knowledge to me and my brothers and sisters. Qualifications for the task seemed unimportant. Miss Easom, though a thoroughly splendid and pleasant person, had been an office worker. Of the four governesses who came to us in nine years only one, Mrs Cornock, was a trained teacher; yet my entire education after the two or three early years in Adelaide was supervised by them. In case it is thought that we were neglected children I should point out that teaching us was the governess's only duty. The other six children then living in Alice Springs did not go to school at all.

Our education came to us as best it could on occasions, but it invariably came. Diversions were few enough to allow ample time for reading and study. Reading, in fact, was one of our chief pleasures. My father subscribed to several national magazines and the operators subscribed to others which were passed around. I read them avidly, and any books I could lay my hands on. Father's best pals were Charles Dickens, William Shakespeare, and Mark Twain. Many roads did I travel with them after my father had rocked himself to sleep in front of the fire and let a book drop. We had no examinations, no exam nerves, and no homework, although there were extra-curricular tasks when Mort and I began to learn drawing by correspondence from the Adelaide School of Design. We were its most distant pupils. Our papers were often in the mails for six weeks before we got replies.

I suppose there were occasions when we "played up" and made life miserable for the governess. I remember that it was especially difficult to concentrate on our work on "Court" days. My father, by virtue of his position as officer in-charge of the telegraph station, had been sworn in as a Special Magistrate and was therefore the most important man in thousands of square miles. In Adelaide, he'd been just another telegraph operator, but here he was an S.M., with all the power that that entailed. His diary records many instances of his having deprived aborigines of their freedom, generally for spearing cattle, and banishing them to Port Augusta for six months. On Court days the station became the hub of Alice Springs, if it wasn't already. Men I'd never seen before arrived from remote cattle stations. Mounted Constable Charles Brookes appeared in his antiquated tight fitting uniform but was such an imposing figure that we regarded him with awe. And there was the usual depressing collection of aboriginal prisoners and witnesses in chains.

The staff dining-room doubled as a Courtroom for the day. As this was next door to the schoolroom it wasn't surprising that our concentration wandered. Prisoners were released from their neck chains one at a time and brought in to be tried. Mounted Constable Brookes was Court crier, prosecutor, and chief Crown witness. He called the case, outlined the facts to the Bench, and then gave evidence to support himself. Generally he was rewarded with a conviction. In this way we heard many interesting sidelights of life in Alice Springs that wouldn't otherwise have come our way—and not all of them concerned aboriginal prisoners. In fact, I remember one white man who appeared as a witness one week and as a prisoner the next.

My father probably knew little more than I did about the law, for he'd never had any experience with it; but I must say that he looked the part, and I was proud of him. His demeanour and physical appearance were just right for a judge—heavily moustached, portly, slightly irritable though supremely dignified while sitting on his Bench (which happened to be the dining-room table), and, above all, eminently fair. He even tried to extend justice to the aborigines and temper it with mercy; at the turn of the century in Central Australia that was not at all an everyday occurrence. As a matter of fact, any white man who demonstrated impartiality in affairs affecting the aborigines was in danger of being branded as a radical. I was especially proud of him when Mounted Constable Brookes addressed him as "Your Honour." To me, aged eight, that was next to "Your Majesty."

My father's diary includes such entries as these:

Feb. 7, 1901: George (alias Nelong) , Tom Cribb and Aralcaringa, aborigines, six months each at Port Augusta gaol.

June 23: Heard ten cases against aborigines at Heavitree Gap gaol. Sentenced each to six months, Port Augusta.

July 18: Corporal Naulty left for Oodnadatta with ten aboriginal prisoners.

August 8: Native charged with stealing beef. Six months at Port Augusta.

But to show that his justice was tempered with mercy, both for humans and animals, there are also these extracts:

Dec. 12, 1901: Sambo broke into store, stole 15 lb. flour, 1 lb. tea, butcher's knife, sugar, etc. I got the goods back, so gave him 5 lb. of flour and cleared him off to go to Barrow Creek.

Oct. 20, 1905: White men Lennon and Gregory fined 7/6d. each camel—11 and 12 camels respectively—for cruelty. Worked camels with sore backs.

Sometimes his diary entries had nothing to do with the law but still reflected compassion:

Jan. 27, 1903: Gave flour to destitute swagmen who had walked 350 miles from Oodnadatta to Winnecke goldfield.

May 6, 1905: Treated sore shoulders of horses with Reckitts Blue, kerosene and unslaked lime.

The tedium was relieved, too, by walkabouts and ride-abouts, talkabouts and singing. During the few short months of winter cold the fire in our dining-room rarely went out. Huge mulga logs were heaved into the fireplace each afternoon by the native boys and our quarters fairly glowed with warmth. It must have been a different matter for the staff in their spartan rooms with cold stone floors, draughty doors, and beds lit by a solitary candle. No wonder they were attracted like moths to the light of our hanging lamp, the matting on our floor, the fireplace, and the fellowship of a young family. We loved them to come, for the price of admission was to be roped for a game of Snakes and Ladders with one of the children, frequently me.

With no homework hanging over our heads, we were carefree and happy. Sing-songs, with the governess playing a piano that had been carried by wagon from Oodnadatta, were one of our favourite diversions. The lamp was taken into the next room and placed on a small central table; the pianos of those days were equipped with brackets to hold two candles and these were lit. With only that illumination, and with the rest of the room in deep shadow, the singers had to get close to the pianist and the song book to follow the words and the music. In nine years, I can't think of one man who didn't singe his eyebrows or a woman who wasn't in danger of being burnt alive. Eight years after our arrival, on my sixteenth birthday, we were still enjoying musical evenings. By that time I was playing the piano myself, having been taught by the governesses. My party guests that night were six older men, all of them smoking pipeful after pipeful of strong tobacco. I don't know how I lived through those thick clouds of smoke, let alone sang through them. A little later Consie sang too, but for a different reason; on her way to bed she found a wild dingo in the room, its eyes glowing green in the light from the candle. Before anyone could get a rifle the dingo escaped through the door and fled.

My brother Mort and I had an equally alarming experience one dark-as-pitch night while walking two miles home after visiting Mrs Charles Meyers in the township. We had come through Middle Park and had almost reached the Todd near the telegraph station when we both became aware of strange soft sounds around us...sighs which might have been caused either by anger or pleasure and may have meant doom for us.

"What's that?" I asked Mort.

"I don't...I don't know," he quavered.

Then I caught the distinctive smell of camels and we realized that a string of them had arrived in our absence to camp there. Though we couldn't see them, they were probably asleep; what concerned us was that if we disturbed one and it rose, the others might stampede. In that event they would assuredly run over the top of us.

Mort and I groped our way to the Todd one foot at a time, terrified of being bitten or trampled to death in the next moment. The camels were bad tempered because their noses had recently been pierced for leadlines; one had rolled on a man and killed him, and we knew that the slightest upset could cause them to rise and trample us. As we reached the bank of the river a shape loomed up directly in front of me and gave a grunt of surprise. Panic-stricken, I gave a wild yell of fear and then—what blessed relief—found that it was one of our camp natives. What he was doing prowling around in the dark I never knew or cared; he was dressed only in an old rag, but I nevertheless clutched the filthy creature thankfully, though at any other time I'd not have gone near him. He seemed equally relieved to find that we were nothing worse than white children; I'm sure he expected that the evil Kadaitcha Man, the tribal executioner, had caught up with him and was about to break his neck.

Subsequently I saw grown men and women at whom the Kadaitcha had "pointed the bone." They were dying of fright, their eyes staring and vacant, some silent, some uttering gibberish, but all refusing to eat and wasting away, completely terrorized by the spell cast upon them by the traditional Doctor Blackfellow.

However, one mustn't blame the camels for being sensitive. They had much to withstand. Apart from having their noses pierced they were driven almost mad by the stings of March flies. Their huge bodies with short tails were ill equipped to deal with tormenting insects. Leslie Spicer, an old friend of telegraph station days, remembers seeing one string of fifty camels all temporarily blinded by March flies. Nevertheless, there were times when camels became a pest. At Marree on one occasion two thousand were shot because they were spoiling the waterholes and denying them to cattle. Another time in the grim early days of the outback three thousand magnificent wild horses were shot there for the same reason.

My other great diversion was to ride horses. Soon after we arrived at Alice Springs I was taught to ride by several of the men on the station. Hacks were plentiful and I had my choice of excellent mounts. When I was still a young girl I was able to ride astride the horse, but when I became "a young lady," aged twelve, this was no longer becoming. I then had to ride side-saddle, a most awkward position which I detested. One had to be very careful not to fall over backwards from the horse, especially when it turned sharply. When that happened one's claims to being elegant and ladylike disappeared rather more quickly than if the display had been prevented by riding astride. However, women have had to suffer worse penalties to preserve the modesty of their sex; I suppose I shouldn't complain about having had to make my contribution.

As my skill increased so did my love of riding until it became my keenest pleasure. The horses were caught and saddled for us by the native horseboys, so that all we had to do was mount and ride away. And what excursions we had! There were no roads to worry us and no traffic. Within a minute of leaving the station we could be in the hills and gullies of the magnificent MacDonnell Ranges, secure always in the knowledge that if we became lost in the bush our horses would take us back home if given their heads. My diary reminds me just how much I enjoyed these outings:

Jan. 3: Rode to Attack Gap (8½ miles) .

Jan. 6: Mort, Consie and I rode to Wigley waterhole. Scarcely any water there but saw three snakes. I rode "Tommy."

Mar. 24: Rode to Emily Creek and through the township.

May 1: My birthday. Rode to a picnic along the Charles River.

Sept. 20: A glorious ride on "Zoe" along the Undoolya road. Rain in our faces, stinging as we rode along.

Dec. 24: Rode out with Mort and Consie to get mistletoe for Christmas. We went up the Charles, then across the plain and around the township.

Dec. 25: Rode up the North "road," then into the township. Didn't see a single white man in the town.

Dec. 31: Glorious ride home from the township in the moonlight. Bright as day. Hills looked very beautiful. Crowd of men sitting around the hotel as we passed; they all cheered us.

This was our equivalent for the young people of today who "go for a burn" in sports cars, perhaps for hundreds of miles. If we covered twenty miles in a day we thought we'd been for a long ride. Once when we drove fifty-two miles in the buggy between dawn and dusk we talked about it for weeks as though we'd just broken some long-standing record.

We were almost equally fond of walking and my diary is full of references to walks through the hills and in to town.

These walkabouts and rideabouts, frequent as they were, weren't as constant as the marathon talkabouts, all in Morse code, that went on day and night in the telegraph office. Having got to Alice Springs in 1899 after a fortnight's buggy ride one might have been excused for boasting about the remoteness of our station. So it was, in a physical and geographic sense. But if the standard of isolation was our proximity to the news of the world from which we were so far removed, then we were not far away at all; in fact we were closer to it than the people in the State capitals.

Every word of world news—the end of the Boer War, the death of Queen Victoria, the San Francisco earthquake, the winner of the Derby—passed through Alice Springs telegraph station on its way from Darwin, where the international cable came ashore, to Adelaide.

Not that we were kept fully informed, either by my father or by the operators. Far from it. Telegraphists are not supposed to divulge any of the information that comes into their hands in the course of their duties. Although that is understandable for matters of a private nature, we thought it was carrying things to absurd lengths that the rules should be so strictly kept in regard to world events. I often felt that my father was bursting with important news that he refused to tell us about, even though it would be published in all Australian papers next day and would thus become public knowledge long before we could have "leaked" it to anyone by the methods of communication open to us. Where his official duty was concerned, however, my father scrupulously observed the regulations. While he and the other operators were mines of topical information, as abreast of the news as they could possibly be, nothing was repeated outside the office unless it involved international tragedy—though why there should have been even that concession I can't imagine. I also couldn't understand why my mother didn't berate him for his secretiveness, but she seemed to accept it patiently. Perhaps she was told privately when we were not listening. Not more than three or four times during our nine years' stay did father break his vow of silence in my presence.

I remember him coming to the house one morning and saying regretfully, "Well, the poor old lady has gone at last." That's how we heard of the death of Queen Victoria.

We were told about the end of the Boer War, in which we had scant interest anyway, and of the great San Francisco earthquake, which made a tremendous stir. Apart from that, we could read all about it when the weekly papers arrived next month.

Alice Springs telegraph station was—and is—what is known as a repeater. Because of the great distance and the comparatively primitive means of transmission when the O.T. Line was first built, all telegraphic signals had to be "boosted" at frequent intervals so that they were strong enough to be read at the receiving end. In the early days the Morse signals were repeated by hand from Alice Springs; that is, every cable, telegram, and Press message was re-transmitted by the Alice Springs operators. With the development of better equipment that was made unnecessary, but the original signal from Darwin still had to be given a kick along. This was done at varying times at Pine Creek, Katherine, Daly Waters, Powell Creek, Tennant Creek, Barrow Creek, Alice Springs, Charlotte Waters, Oodnadatta, Marree, and Port Augusta. Today all messages are boosted six times between Darwin and Alice Springs—at Pine Creek, Katherine, Larrimah, Newcastle Waters, Tennant Creek, and Barrow Creek—but it involves nothing more than pressing a switch on highly technical equipment.

Under certain atmospheric conditions, especially in damp weather, there was a danger that leakages of current might cause the signals to be dissipated. Instead of reaching Alice Springs in good order they might disappear for ever somewhere in the lands of the Warramunga tribesmen, who could read neither Morse nor English. To avoid that needed constant vigilance by the telegraphists at repeating stations, of which we were one. Four operators were therefore needed to monitor the traffic day and night. The telegraphists also had to maintain the batteries—about five hundred of them—which gave us the power to boost the signals. The batteries consisted of wet cells, each with a large glass jar containing a solution of water and magnesia and a lead and zinc plate. Fitting neck-down into the top of each jar was a bottle containing copper sulphate, commonly known as bluestone. A small glass tube in the cork of the bottle allowed drops of copper sulphate to fall on the lead plate, which gradually became coated with copper. Insulated wires from the zinc and copper enabled the hundreds of cells to be linked together, thus generating a constant supply of power. Every few months the batteries were recharged with the addition of new copper.

Although I lived within hopping distance of those batteries

for nine years, I seldom entered the building which housed them. It was not forbidden to us; it was simply that in those days girls were thought to be unladylike if they interested themselves in anything more complicated than dressmaking. I knew that one of the buildings was called the battery room but I shunned it like an aboriginal would shun a caveful of evil spirits. In fact, I had to seek the help of Leslie Spicer, one of the operators who was there in our time, before being able to explain here how they worked. We were then still far removed from the day when girls would qualify as mechanics and pilots and operate complicated electronic equipment. I was equally disinterested in the normal postal and telegraph duties and the ceaseless reporting of meteorological observations. I could never understand why someone in Adelaide would want to know the Alice Springs temperature, rate of evaporation, strength of winds and density of clouds every four hours, day and night. But they did, and this was a service supplied by the operator on duty. I know now, of course, that this information was vital in establishing a weather picture for men who would forecast what conditions might be expected.

One part of the station's inventory interested me more than any other. This was the mob of about sixty beautiful horses from which, more or less, I could choose my own hack. They grazed along the river bank west of the station, but seldom roamed more than six or seven miles away, although there was scarcely a fence worthy of the name between them and Port Augusta.

Why should a telegraph station need such a large "plant" of horses? The fact is that the O.T. Line couldn't have remained open without them; for more than fifty years after it was built horses provided the transport for the operators and linemen who went out in blistering heat and perishing cold, year in and year out, whenever a fault was reported.

Every day about thirty horses were brought in by the aboriginal horseboy and yarded. Next day they were released and a fresh mob yarded. They had to be available at the shortest notice in case of a break or a fault in the telegraph line. When that happened an operator with an aboriginal left from each of the two stations between which the fault had occurred. One rode north and the other south until the trouble was found. After long periods of experimentation, my father discovered a means of locating a breakdown within a few miles, thus saving two parties going out. This was done by measuring the resistance in the wire to signals sent along it. His discovery was a most important one in helping to speed the correction of faults and thus restore international communications, but he got no acknowledgement for it. However, the time that elapsed before restoration could be made was still governed by the speed of a horse.

Repairing the line must have been a frightful job, especially in summer when conditions were barely tolerable in temperatures ranging up to 150 degrees and perhaps higher. There was little shade on the track; in any case, the operator had to keep going, frequently spending several days in the saddle in heat which had to be experienced to be realized. Little wonder that the operators were pleased when this duty was taken over by linemen.

I have an old letter of Leslie Spicer's, written from Barrow Creek, which gives some idea of what a breakdown meant for the man who had to repair it. He wrote:

> On Christmas Day I received word that the line was down south of Barrow Creek. The lineman was suffering from sunstroke from an earlier trip, so I closed the office at nine o'clock and rode out myself to repair the damage. That night my black boy and I camped under the shadow of Central Mt. Stuart, the geographic centre of the continent about forty miles from Barrow Creek. You can imagine what the heat was like there in mid-summer(We started next morning at about three o'clock to cover

as many miles as possible before the sun got up. We found the fault at eleven o'clock, thirty-five miles from our night camp. A few miles further on we removed a second fault and then rode to Mt. Boothby, near Aileron, to camp. This was ninety miles from Barrow Creek. In the morning we rode a few miles further south to make sure there were no broken insulators in the vicinity and then turned for home, reaching Barrow Creek late next day. I had hardly had time for a bath when one of the lines went wrong again! At dawn we were once more in the saddle, riding south, and found- the fault near Tea Tree Well, fifty miles away. The last four miles of this ride took us nearly three hours because one of the horses was badly staked and could scarcely walk. I would not have troubled to go on but I knew there were two white men at Tea Tree who could help me get the splinter from the horse's foot. I re-opened the Barrow Creek office four days after leaving. Three hours later word came through that the lines were again twisted about midway to Alice Springs. Now I had enjoyed my ten hours daily in the saddle, though some folk would say that five miles an hour was irksome. All the same, I'd had enough of the flies and the sun, which had scorched my hands until they were raw, so I went on strike. There was a line-party at Alice Springs. At my request they drove out in a buggy and restored communications two days later.

My father's diary shows that he, too, drove out on inspection trips, sometimes with the weather at the opposite extreme. I'm not sure that his task was any less arduous than that of the linemen in summer. In May 1904, for instance, he left home on a trip to Barrow Creek. With him in the buggy (as an officer-in-charge he travelled in style) was Harry Kunoth, a man of

German descent with many years' experience in Central Australia. His descendants, of whom the coloured film star Ngarla Kunoth was one (she played the lead role in Jedda), are still living there today.

My father records that on 23rd May he and Kunoth were stranded by heavy rain which made the ground so soft that the horses couldn't pull the buggy through the bog. That night and the two following nights they slept in the buggy with a tarpaulin rigged over it to run off as much of the rain as possible. I've never tried sleeping in a buggy but I imagine it's not the most comfortable bed, especially under those conditions.

On 26th May they were able to move again but soon ran into a bog. They had to unload the buggy, carry their load across, and then build a "road" of bushes to give the wheels a chance of turning. That done, they took hold of the shafts and lent their man-power to the horse-power in hauling the buggy out of difficulties. They were out of meat. One evening a wild turkey flew against the wire and fell dead between father and Harry Kunoth. It was promptly plucked, boiled, and eaten.

> May 26: What a fearful day!
>
> May 27: Reached Tea Tree Well, 120 miles from Alice Springs. [He had been five days getting there, or 24 miles a day.] Bitterly cold wind. Spoke to the family at night.

And I have a note in my diary for that day to remind me that it was a Sunday evening, that we were having tea before a log fire, and that we were all wonderfully comfortable. Then there is this comment: "Father sounded very forlorn."

Sixty years later, one is scarcely surprised. A telegraph lineman who was asked to go out under such conditions today would probably resign on the spot.

But how did my father sound forlorn? How could we hear him when the only means of communication I have mentioned has been the Morse telegraph? The fact is that my father had a private telephone. This was an unheard of luxury in those days—to such an extent that the government which owned a telegraph line across Australia thought it unnecessary and an unwarranted expense to equip the staff with telephones. If a postmaster or an operator wanted the convenience of a phone he had to buy it himself, and that's what my father had done. When he did so, perhaps he had in mind just such a situation as that which arose on that May night when I was thirteen years old. Frozen, forlorn, and far from home, he "tapped" the line and spoke to his family. I think this was the first time I ever heard a telephone conversation. They were so rare that in our nine years at Alice Springs I can remember the first occasion when the Alice Springs staff spoke to the Darwin staff by means other than the telegraph. Periodically, when the line was free of telegraph traffic, there were brief conversations between the Alice Springs and Barrow Creek staffs; but that was also so infrequent that when it happened it was a matter for comment.

Today a telephonist in Darwin can dial any number in Adelaide or Brisbane, both two thousand miles away, without the assistance of other telephonists at the receiving end. She can also dial numbers in South Australian country towns like Port Augusta, Balaklava, and Port Pirie. I'm sure my father didn't imagine in his wildest dreams that such impersonal miracles would eventually be happening on his beloved O.T. Line. But they tell me there are bigger and better miracles still to come—it won't be long, I'm assured, before I can pick up my telephone and dial any number in Australia. And my grandchildren will probably be able to dial any number in the world. My father might not have felt so badly about the weather on that winter's night if he had known this would happen in such a relatively short time...

May 28: Stuck at Skull Creek. [Shades of Blackfellows' Bones.] Road one giant sea of mud up to the horses' bellies. A packhorse went down, with only its head and neck visible.

Kunoth had to strip his clothes off and cut the pack off the horse. After a lot of trouble we got him out. Several other horses had narrow escapes. We saw two belonging to a droving party. It was impossible to extricate them from the mud and they had been shot to release them from their suffering.

May 29: Decided to try to get through. After a short distance the horses went down again. One took a lot of time and trouble to get up. Unloaded buggy and carried our equipment through. Then three blackboys, Kunoth and self manhandled the buggy to firmer ground. Later we came to a white man's camp. He was dead in the bush. I tapped the line and told the police.

How does this appeal to you now as you pick up your telephone and dial the number for the interstate or international exchange? How does it appeal as you sit behind the steering wheel of your car, with the speedometer needle flicking around sixty miles an hour, the tyres humming uniformly on the bitumen road? Alice Springs to Barrow Creek now takes about three hours by road. Aeroplanes leave the Alice and the pilot tells the passengers that Barrow Creek can be seen on the left—just half an hour later. My father took eight days in a buggy, and was away for so long that rations for the return trip had to be taken out to him by Jim Raka, an aboriginal employed at our station. He noted the distance and time taken for each of his trips, like this: Today's distance 39 miles, time 8 hours = average 5 miles an hour...Distance 40 miles, time 10 hours = average 4 miles an hour.

In spite of the annoyance, the inconvenience, and the discomfort when things went wrong, the Line was our best friend. It was our one link with civilization in the event of sickness or accident, even though we knew that any help we called in an emergency would arrive much too late. There were no aeroplanes, and therefore no flying doctor services; no radio, and therefore no rescue at all for people who lived away from the Line; yet it was comforting to know that the two wires running from the Arafura Sea to the Southern Ocean, stretching straight ahead through gibber plains and sandhills, through wide creek beds, mulga scrub, and great rocky ranges, on and on through the Empty Land...well, we were pleased they were there, if only to tell our friends that we were in trouble.

Here I've been writing about the unimagined improvement that has been made in communications since then; yet the difference in our day to what it once was must have been just as great. It seems difficult to believe that before the O.T. Line spanned the continent the only link Australia had with the rest of the world was by ship, the nearest cable station being at Java. The "singing strings," as we sometimes called the Line, and the extension of the cable to Darwin, changed all that. Messages could then be exchanged between Australia and England in a few hours—in minutes if necessary. It never occurred to us, therefore, remote and isolated as we were, that we didn't live in the most modern of all worlds. Indeed, at that time, we did.

Perhaps I'm prejudiced, but I believe the O.T. Line contributed as much to the development of the nation as any other single factor. It stimulated trade. British commercial enterprise could have a daily report on market situations and was thus encouraged to invest in a stable and growing country, although it was then still a group of separate and diverse colonies. At first it was all done on one iron wire stretching for two thousand miles; later that was duplicated with a copper wire. For the young colony of South Australia, with a population of less than quarter of a million people, it was a tremendous and courageous undertaking to attempt stringing poles and wires across a hostile land that had been traversed for the first time only eight years earlier. The story of how it was done, of how the problems and difficulties were overcome, is one of drama and romance unsurpassed in the nation's history.

Nevertheless, when we were there, although it had been built less than thirty years earlier, it was taken for granted. Only long after I returned to Adelaide did I hear the story of how it was built and of the problems which faced the plucky men who strung the wires through an unknown and often waterless wilderness.

Interstate jealousies had been overcome. Queensland had competed strongly with South Australia but withdrew from the race when it was found to be more practicable to bring the Line from Port Darwin, where the cable from East Java was to come ashore, through Central Australia to Adelaide.

For two reasons South Australia was vitally interested in having the Line pass through its territory. The first was to earn transit revenue on all cable messages to the eastern colonies via Adelaide. The second was to open direct overland communication with its sub-colony in the tropical north, which had been transferred to it less than ten years earlier.

In 1870 the British-Australian Telegraph Company signed an agreement with South Australia to lay a cable from East Java to Port Darwin on condition that a landline was built over the gap of 1,800 miles between Port Augusta and Port Darwin, then a tiny settlement.

The landline and the sea cable were both to be opened before 1st January, 1872. This left barely eighteen months in which to complete what was then a vast undertaking. The contracts included penalty clauses for delays or nonfulfilment. Looking back to our buggy drive from Oodnadatta, I can appreciate the courage of men who signed contracts without intimate knowledge of the difficulties they were likely to encounter.

Our transport. Passengers, Donnell and Edna; driver Jack, watched by Consie and Mort

The family and white staff just before we left Alice Springs in 1908

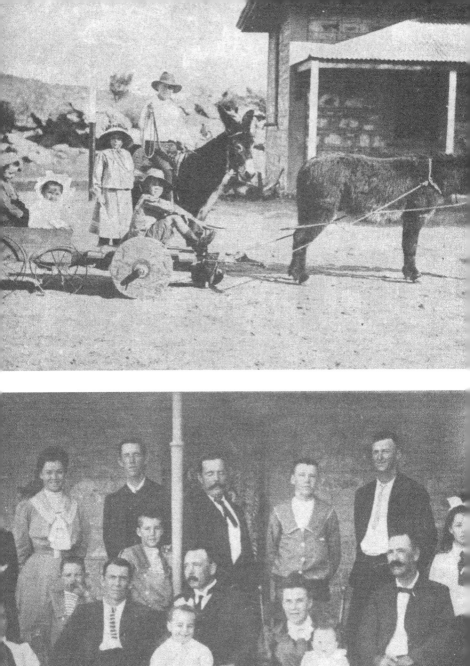
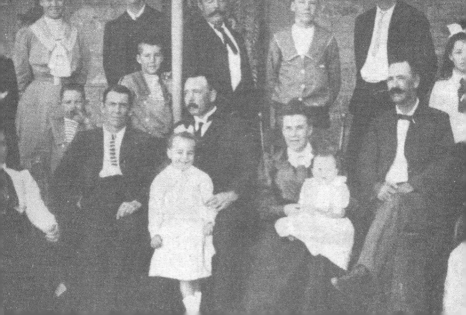

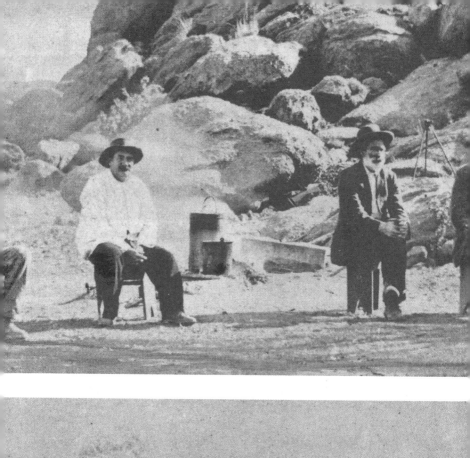

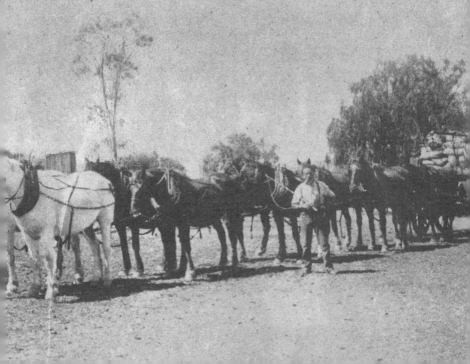

John McDouall Stuart had shown that a land corridor through the Centre was possible but he had also shown that it was possible only at the cost of supreme effort under conditions which were cruel and often barely tolerable. Even with Stuart's reports, almost nothing was known of the country north of the Salt Lakes. To say the least, men who contracted to build a telegraph line in these circumstances were gambling with their luck.

The South Australian Parliament passed a bill authorizing the expenditure of £120,000 on the project, an amount fully in keeping with the traditional parsimony of governments. Perhaps it did reflect optimism that the job could be done quickly and cheaply, in spite of an estimate that the cost would be not less than £338,000. In any case, the important thing was to have the work begun, for when that happened the Government would be committed to completing it.

The South Australian Postmaster-General, Mr Charles Todd, was made responsible for the overall construction. The O.T. Line is his memorial as much as anyone's. He showed a great flair for organization and kept the work going when it seemed inevitable that it must break down.

Todd divided the route into three roughly equal sections of six hundred miles each, to be worked simultaneously. The southern section to the Macumba River, north of Oodnadatta, was completed on time without mishap. The going was comparatively easy and communications were good, although there was then no railway north of Port Augusta.

For the central section of 621 miles from north of Macumba to Tennant Creek the lines of communication began to be

O.T. Line maintenance party. From left: George Hablett and Albert Hewish, G. Ross

George Hablett with a 10-horse team, wagon, and stores

extended. All provisions and supplies—the posts, the wire, the insulators, the food—had to be carried in horsedrawn vehicles or on the backs of camels.

South of Darwin on the northern section, especially during the tropical "wet" season, the difficulties were still worse, and it was here that the longest delays occurred, although they had been anticipated in the central section. Contractors were so wary of the Macumba—Tennant Creek leg that it was decided to build it with five separate parties of government employees.

How much did the Government pay for the Line? On the southern section, for more than 500 miles north from Port Augusta, the rate was £41 a mile. The successful tenderer was Mr E. M. Bagot.

The rate for the northern section varied. For the first forty miles from Port Darwin it was only £39 a mile. From there for the next 250 miles it was £60 a mile. Then it rose to £89 a mile, and the last 100 miles to the 19th parallel just north of Tennant Creek was £92 a mile.

John Ross went out from Port Augusta ahead of the construction parties. Surveyors were with him to chart the route, much of which amounted to nothing less than exploration of an unknown land. But they were the men who let daylight in to Central Australia and it was this advance party, and John Ross in particular, who established the site for Alice Springs. In due course it became an advanced supply depot.

On 7th July, 1870, Charles Todd gave Ross a letter of appointment stipulating that he was to be paid £450 a year for this extremely onerous task. If that should be thought a miserly sum, Todd also instructed that the wages of three labourers Ross was to take with him "must not exceed 21/- a week."

Ross had three prime objects in selecting a route: it had to give easy access to timber suitable for poles twenty feet long and ten inches in diameter at the butt, to permanent water, and to country free from inundations and suitable for sinking holes four feet deep.

From what I saw of it, he must have had a difficult task in all respects. Todd, nevertheless, instructed Ross to be quick about it and to give him detailed reports and survey maps within three months, and reminded him that his services were subject to termination on one month's notice.

I've no doubt that at times Todd was forced to become something of a bullock driver, but much more than his personal reputation depended on the successful outcome of what was then one of the biggest undertakings ever attempted in Australia. Present-day contractors, equipped with all sorts of mechanical devices, would turn grey if faced with the problems that Todd had to overcome. On the central section, for instance, the five government parties had 165 horses, 210 bullocks, and 100 men who had to be fed and supplied. Their transport consisted of fifteen horse wagons, seventeen bullock drays, one bullock wagon, and five "express" wagons, whatever they might have been. In addition, a Mr Harley Bacon was put in charge of a receiving and forwarding depot on the Finke River (generally dry) which had no fewer than two thousand sheep. To me it is little short of miraculous that those sheep managed to cross hundreds of miles of boiling gibber plains.

The men who worked on the central section are well remembered in place names throughout the Northern Territory today. I'm sure nobody will dispute their right to that kind of immortality. They included R. R. Knuckey, Christopher Giles, G. R. McMinn, C. Musgrave, W. W. Mills, A. G. Burt, A. T. Woods, S. Jarvis, W. Harvey, and J. L. Roberts. The party led by Harvey left Adelaide on 5th September, 1870, but did not reach its base at latitude south 21 degrees, north of Barrow Creek, until 24th May, 1871. Seven days later they planted their first pole.

Contractors working on the northern section of the line had underestimated the effect of the tropical monsoon on the transport of material and men by horse-drawn vehicles. The first pole was planted near Darwin in September 1870, and within 54 days 89 miles of line had been built. By January 1871 it had reached Katherine River, more than 200 miles away. But then the skies opened and the men were hopelessly isolated from their base. A contract let to Darwent and Dalwood was declared void, and a fresh expedition under the command of the Assistant Engineer-in-Chief, R. C. Patterson, was sent around the continent in six vessels. It included 200 men, 170 horses, and 500 bullocks. Patterson's expedition arrived at Darwin during the hot dry months immediately preceding another "wet" season. The country was bare of feed and long dry stages had to be covered.

Before wells could be sunk and material carted inland a monsoon of remarkable intensity was upon them and all work stopped again. Severe losses of stock were sustained, including about forty per cent of the bullocks. Patterson had to go by boat to Normanton, in northern Queensland, and thence to the nearest telegraph station at Gilbert River to call for help.

Todd himself went to the rescue with three ships and more men and established a base on the Roper River. But nothing could be done until the country dried out sufficiently to make movement possible.

Work began again in April 1872, and all sections were finally joined on 22nd August, 1872. Meanwhile, however, Todd established a horse-express to carry messages across the gap, which at first was 262 miles wide. In what had become a race against time to complete the England-Australia cable link, the South Australian Government saved considerable face while the horse-express was operating because of a cable fault between Darwin and Java, which wasn't repaired for several weeks. But when the ends met at Frew's Ponds, near

Newcastle Waters, on 22nd August, Charles Todd received congratulatory messages from all over the world and was able to report that the Australian colonies at long last were connected with the grand electric chain which united all the nations of the earth.

That, they thought, was that. But it wasn't. Allowance had not been made for the voracious appetites and the menacing mandibles of countless millions of white ants. Even before the line was finished some of the wooden poles were showing signs of being eaten away. While men, animals, and equipment were still in the area it was decided to replace them with iron poles. Thousands of them had to be brought from England. The original cost of £338,000 was thus increased to £480,000. It must have hurt badly but the young South Australian colony refused outside financial help. Until the great industrial progress of the post-war years the more affluent States were inclined to be critical and patronizing of what they regarded as a backward neighbour. But they have never been able to contest that it was South Australia alone which gave them the international communications to make commercial enterprise possible. It was a courageous act by a relatively poor colony and one that is seldom appreciated.

Chapter Five

DOCTOR BLACKFELLOWS

AS TIME PASSED, OUR INTEREST IN THE THINGS around us, notably the telegraph line, was replaced by a deeper interest in the aboriginal people. We were not allowed to visit their camps on the river bank, so my youthful study of them was restricted to the men, women, and children who came to the station for food or treatment of their ills. And there was never any shortage of them.

The Aranda had had only thirty years of spasmodic contact with Europeans. The majority were still primitive, naked nomads who hunted their food and lived by tribal laws that had been handed down orally through thousands of years, for they had no written language. Even among the people living around the station there had been little progress towards the kind of sophistication that some have achieved today. They did not understand the most rudimentary principles of hygiene. They slept on the ground with dogs, and ate food with their fingers. Seldom did I see one of them washing his body; that would have been regarded as wanton waste of water in a land where there was frequently not enough to drink. Although this was all quite abhorrent to me, I was aware of the reasons, which I had to admit seemed sensible; but when I occasionally came face to face with some of their other practices I was utterly repelled.

One of the few occasions when I visited the camp, or its vicinity, was with my mother. I accompanied her one evening on an errand of mercy to take invalid food to Tom, an aboriginal employed as horse-tailer at the station. Tom had suddenly been stricken with an illness that could not be diagnosed and his condition was rapidly deteriorating. We found him lying on the ground some distance from the camp. A filthy old Medicine Man was in attendance beside him and appeared to be looking very pleased with his efforts. And well he might. Spread out before him he had an imposing array of pebbles, pieces of wood, and other odds and ends, all of which, he assured us, he'd sucked from various parts of Tom's anatomy. With a ponderousness that would not have been out of place in a Harley Street specialist, he made us understand that he had got to the root of Tom's trouble and that the patient was as good as cured. Tom seemed equally confident about his recovery. He was able to communicate freely with us, having been taught to speak excellent English by Mr Gillen, my father's predecessor. He was an intelligent and likeable man who had adopted white men's habits and put on their clothing. Reconciling that with his utter gullibility in other matters was therefore difficult. It is noteworthy, however, that sixty years later, after much closer contact with white people than was possible at the time, many of the Aranda hold as strongly to their practices as they did then. The power of the Doctor Blackfellows, and of malevolent Kadaitcha Men, is an indisputable fact. Bone-pointing is as effective now as it was before European settlement and will probably remain so until these primitive people absorb a much deeper personal knowledge of anatomy.

As a final flourish to impress us, the old Medicine Man sucked Tom's arm and slyly produced a jagged piece of broken glass. Both he and Tom looked shocked when Mother hinted that the glass could not possibly have been inside Tom's body as the old scamp insisted. In any case, Tom assured her that he felt much better and would soon be able to attend to his duties again. A few days later he was dead, apparently the victim of a man whose ability to cause death by auto-suggestion was superior to that of the Doctor Blackfellow to circumvent it with similar hocuspocus.

Tom's was the first death to occur on the station since our arrival and was the cause of our introduction to a period of the most mournful wailing I had ever heard. It was eerie and depressing but unmistakably sincere, and that always seemed to be so after subsequent deaths. Those tribesmen and women who didn't feel sufficiently upset by a relative's death soon produced that result by cutting their heads and bodies with stones and sharp sticks until the blood ran in torrents. Sometimes the wailing from the river bank continued all night; later when I saw some of the self-inflicted wounds, often deep gashes up to six inches long, I wasn't at all surprised.

The influence of the Doctor Blackfellows in our midst was profound. The mere mention of their names was enough to strike terror into the hearts of most of the men and women with whom we had daily contact. Since the first anthropologists went among the aborigines to study their lives and customs, they have been puzzled by the ability of these so-called Medicine Men to cause death by psychic means and of others to prevent it. What has been so startling in many cases is that there has been no apparent physical cause of the victim's death, and nothing that has been done by skilled European doctors has reversed the process once it has begun. Medical practitioners have cured sick aborigines of all the symptoms of their illnesses, and yet been unable to restore their patients to health, thus concluding that there is something unfathomable in the natives' attitude towards sickness which can only be cured psychologically. But that is not always successful either; Tom was convinced that he would get better, which was generally a good sign, and yet we had this fearful wailing to prove that he was dead.

One of the apparent disadvantages of the pointing-sticks used by some Medicine Men was that their evil influence could rub off accidentally. Anyone who got too near to the flames, so to speak, would be burnt. During his term at the telegraph station, Mr Gillen collaborated with Professor Sir Baldwin Spencer in anthropological research and the subsequent publication of *The Native Tribes of Central Australia*, which is still regarded by academics as the most authoritative text-book on the subject. They reported that one old Medicine Man, after much persuasion, was induced to demonstrate how a particular type of pointing-stick was used. Another native who was with them promptly retired to a distance he considered safe from the death-dealing rays of the stick. The Medicine Man himself, after jerking the stick in a proper manner towards an imaginary victim, said he was rather upset because some of the evil magic had entered his own head. He only gradually regained his equanimity after he was assured that Spencer and Gillen's medicine chest contained sufficient magic to counteract that in the pointing-stick. The old man's chief worry was that he had not made and "sung" the stick himself, and so he did not know exactly what magic was in it.

In case this is thought to be far-fetched, it should be remembered that there are numerous cases of death by auto-suggestion among the aborigines in recent times. Nothing indicates that they have any less fear of Medicine Men now than they had last century or a thousand years ago.

Our aboriginal housemaids were frequently sorry sights after a death in the camp, bringing their dolorous grief into the house and making us feel wretched too. In accordance with tradition, they never mentioned the deceased's name except as "that dead-feller," or by identifying him with a woman, a child, or a particular country. This is a precautionary measure against an age-old belief that the sound of a dead person's name might encourage his spirit to return to the scene to haunt the survivors. It was therefore difficult to establish quickly the names of some of the deceased.

The aborigines made no attempt to forsake their tribal life, and we did not try to interfere except to bring them what help we could. Both my father and mother were constantly "doctoring" sick people. My father kept a separate "medical" diary in which were listed the symptoms and treatment for everything from Acidity to Yaws. It was alphabetically indexed—"Belly, pains in"; "Eyes, granulated," etc.—and scrupulously followed. I have the diary beside me now. The frontispiece consists of printed instructions from the Government Gazette of 1st December, 1896, for the treatment of various poisons. Thus I know that there was no reliable antidote for strychnine, prussic acid, phosphorus, castor oil seeds, and a few other things, although I find that raw eggs are supposed to be good for carbolic acid, and barley water and powdered chalk for oxalic acid. In cases where emetics were recommended we were advised to help induce vomiting by tickling the back of the throat with a feather. There was an intriguing footnote to it all: "The antidotes are such as may be generally used, but in all serious cases of poisoning the earliest attendance of a medical man should be obtained." Just how soon we might have obtained one when the nearest was at Oodnadatta and the only method of travel was by buggy is a matter for conjecture.

In these days of penicillin, sulfa, and other so-called "wonder" drugs, it is interesting to see with what aids my parents attended to the ills of their own family and the big auxiliary family of aborigines. The cure-alls then included glycerine, lime water, castor oil and olive oil, laudanum, carbolic acid, iodine, pulverized charcoal (for foul breath)

, quinine, bismuth, aconite, pulverized rhubarb, essence of ginger (for disordered stomach) , and Fuller's Earth.

Chafes were to be treated with sugar of lead, dandruff with sulphuric acid and lard, toothache with liquid ammonia or oil of cloves, and sunstroke with plain cold water held to the head and chest (though I'm not sure where we were supposed to get cold water when the temperature was 115 degrees in a land without ice or refrigerators) . Digitalis was prescribed for all manner of ills including piles, and bunions could apparently be relieved with a mixture of honey and borax.

My brother Mort became ill with whooping cough in 1900. That must have been a worrying time for my parents, and the medical diary contains many references to the treatment he was given, all of it prescribed by doctors who went to the telegraph office in Adelaide to receive symptoms sent in Morse code by my father. Complications set in during convalescence, including acute itching, ulcerated mouth, blurred vision, swollen glands, upset stomach, and difficulty in swallowing. For this a Dr Michie telegraphed his prescription from Adelaide: A dose of castor oil, then fourhourly doses of chlorate of potash, belladonna, and syrup, plus hot fomentations. Instead of getting better, poor Mort developed diphtheritic paralysis and was very ill for three months, which perhaps isn't surprising.

But the patients in my parents' care were predominantly aboriginal. The fact that neither my father nor my mother had any medical training was of little concern to them, and they came in search of treatment for the smallest complaint—and often for none at all. Men who stoically bore the pain of spear and waddy wounds wanted "rubbin' medicine" and "binjie medicine" at the first sign of an unexplained ache. When there was obviously nothing seriously wrong with them they settled happily enough for cough medicine or something else equally harmless, although nothing was given away needlessly except in minute quantities; always at the back of my father's mind in such cases was the knowledge that everything expended had to be replenished on a camel's back.

Sometimes sick aboriginal women prescribed for themselves, especially when mother was puzzled what to give them. They took good care to see that this self-inflicted treatment was a treat instead. Rice had been their Properly-Number-One-Tucker since the arrival of white men thirty years before. They preferred it to almost anything else. So that when my mother was at a loss about what to do with a sick Lubra, she was often advised by the patient, "Tink'it rice make'im good-feller." But rice was one of the last of our commodities likely to be used for medicine; it was bulky and weighed heavily and could not be given in capsule form, or simply with water added to a tincture. Every grain of it came a thousand miles from Adelaide and was used sparingly as part of our staple diet. Nevertheless, the natives did have great feasts of rice which mother cooked for them. On "rice nights" the women lined up at the kitchen in force, armed with "jampeters," or jam tins, and shouted gleefully as they received their ration. The tins were emptied quickly by delighted children, and the mothers often tried for a second helping.

I was horrified at the pitiful attempts the lubras made at cooking civilized food. They had no idea how to convert flour and water into edible Johnny-cakes or damper; instead, they made a gooey paste which could have been used as an adhesive and ate it with their fingers—uncooked. Once when natural game was scarce during a long drought, and the native hunters often came home empty-handed, my mother had to come to the rescue of dozens of piccaninnies who were near to starvation. Through the worst of the drought she made damper for them every day. In the late afternoon, having roasted herself over a wood stove, she called the piccaninnies to her in fun: "Chook! Chook! Chook!" They ran from all directions, taking their "tucker" greedily and more often than not without a word of thanks, which they didn't understand. When rice was on the menu—and somehow they always seemed to find out in advance—they came even more quickly and fought for a good position in the line.

Curry was a great favourite with the adults and the hotter it was the better they liked it. I have found in my diary a record of one Christmas dinner which the Aranda had from my father: it was a curry made of goat's meat, twenty pounds of rice, and all the apparent left-overs in the storeroom—those items like chutney and dried fruit which were not too popular in the staff kitchen. The curry was made in an enormous cast-iron boiler which seemed to contain enough for a regiment. In any case, it was shared by about two hundred natives who used all manner of utensils, from wooden pitchis to "jampeters" to carry away their ration. I'll never forget that one old man without an adequate dish came along with his filthy hat; it had been lying in the dirt around his camp for months, but that seemed not to worry him. On the contrary, he was glad to have such a commodious container and highly delighted when my mother filled it for him. If the rice was a little weevily after months of storage it represented added flavour for the natives.

There was also coffee, and cake and sweets which mother made for the children. This was all a rare luxury for them, so I'm sure it was the chief means by which the Aranda became impressed with the importance of our Christmas festival.

Three decades earlier Christmas Day was just another hunting day in their lives and invariably a hot one. By the time of our arrival, however, it had become a day of rest for all hands—all, that is, except my mother and father, who worked to feed everyone. They were so exhausted, in fact, that our own Christmas dinner had to be postponed until the evening when they'd have a chance of enjoying it themselves. This devotion to aboriginal welfare on Christmas Day was common to most

European stations and settlements, even in those places where Christian brotherhood and the Golden Rule were not exactly daily observances. Men whose treatment of the natives otherwise bordered on the barbaric seemed unable to resist the Christmas message and extended generous hands filled with food.

This was especially welcome on the Christmas Day that preceded the twentieth century by only one week; for that was ushered in by one of the worst droughts in the history of Central Australia. The phrase "the blacks died like flies" had an awful significance for us all that year, for they did just that. Men, women, and children struggled across unknown deserts to reach the infant civilization they had previously shunned in the hope that they might find survival. Those who reached it did survive, but there were many—hundreds, perhaps thousands—who died in tormented groups around dry waterholes in a land which had long since ceased to provide enough food for their natural game. They ate rats and lizards, dogs and cats—and yet they died. It was a dismal period; I remember that drought hanging oppressively over us all. Our sheep were so poor that a leg of mutton didn't have enough meat to feed our family. We had a concoction known as "Drought Pudding"—a blancmange which my mother renamed because six cows and fifty goats yielded so little milk between them that it had to be made with condensed milk.

Father went to the storeroom every Saturday morning to distribute the natives' rations. Although they had no calendar and apparently understood little about the division of time, they knew without fail when Saturday came. My father's visits to the storeroom on other days of the week passed unnoticed; but his arrival there on Saturdays coincided with that of an assortment of ladies of all ages and sizes carrying tins of all ages and sizes from discarded pepper tins to kerosene tins. When he opened the storeroom door and said "Quei"—the aboriginal word for woman or girl—they burst through with all the excitement of more sophisticated women at bargain-basement sales in a big city store. Though everyone got exactly the same rations of flour, tea, sugar, and tobacco, there was always a scramble to be first served—to get the pick of the crop. The women never seemed to understand that quantities which filled a billycan would scarcely touch the sides in a kerosene tin. Those with smaller tins smiled smugly at my father's generous portions, but the owners of quarter-filled kerosene tins grumbled openly; they would look inside the tin, point to its emptiness, and with wrathful glances reproach my father for his favouritism. When some of the chronic old grumblers lingered on, hoping he would have a change of heart, he'd open the window behind the store and shout "Wei"—their word for men or boys. On that command, the women scattered as though the place had caught fire. Within a few seconds every quei was out of sight and the weis were in full possession.

My father had learnt a few tricks of the trade. He knew, for instance, that under the tribal law certain women were not allowed to look at certain men, nor the men at the women. Tribal law was then still paramount, and kinship avoidance was practised as though their lives depended on it.

The strictest taboo, even today, is that between a man and his mother-in-law. Under the system of promissory marriages that they observe, this can become operative from the moment a girl is born and promised to a certain man. One effect of this law is that it prevents the possibility of competition between a girl and her mother for the affection, of the same man—a very real danger where so often the wife is much younger than the husband and the husband and mother-in-law are of the same age. They must therefore neither speak to nor see one another, and the Aranda, in our day, took great care to ensure that it didn't happen. Kinship avoidance extended to certain blood relationships as well; it was not surprising, in these circumstances, that the women scattered like frightened fowls when the men were summoned.

These taboos caused difficulties when housegirls were being engaged by my mother. After a few months' work, the lubras inevitably came to her with the news that they were leaving.

"Quei, me knock up Tonga work, me go walkabout now," I'd hear them say, and then, as an afterthought, "Might-be Polly come here and work, I reckon."

In this situation my mother had learnt to be careful so as not to upset the tribal sensitivities.

"Very well," she'd say, "but is it all right for Polly to look along Mick?"

Mick, at that time, was the water boy. His duty was to keep the 200-gallon tank on our veranda filled with water carted in buckets from a soakage in the river 100 yards away. If Mick was taboo to the girls there was a daily commotion in the house. Every time he came into view, carrying his buckets on a yoke, the girls dashed for cover and stayed in hiding until he was out of sight again. On the first few occasions, this might have been funny; after that it became irritating, but there was nothing my mother could do to avoid it. On one occasion a temporary housegirl who was caught by surprise at the arrival of the water carrier ran into the kitchen as though she'd seen a ghost and dived under my mother's skirt. Nor would she emerge until assured that the man had gone.

In this respect washing days were generally bedlam, for then extra women came from the camp to help with the family wash. The tubs were adjacent to the tank on the veranda so that every quarter of an hour, with the arrival of the water-boy, most of the washerwomen beat a fast retreat while others not under taboo carried on. I often thought that the girls all rather enjoyed the excitement and treated it as a huge joke, like children playing hide-and-seek. I was sometimes surprised that the washing got done at all. Our unfortunate water boy with more than the usual number of female relatives and potential mothers-in-law seemed to be forever dodging women, and all the women were constantly alert for his arrival. The arbitrary kinship rule made it necessary for him to avoid not only the women in our kitchen but in the staff kitchen as well. As the staff quarters were between our veranda and the river he had almost to circumnavigate the station boundary on each trip, while remaining constantly alert to avoid a face he shouldn't see. I think the poor man was very happy when my father became aware of his predicament and relieved him of that duty.

Clothing the multitude was a task almost as onerous as feeding them. When John McDouall Stuart and John Ross first crossed the MacDonnell Ranges in the 1860s and 1870 the aborigines they saw were entirely naked. But it didn't take long for them to put on white men's cast-off clothes, and though the result was generally a travesty of sartorial elegance it served two purposes.

The first of these was a concession to the white man's prudery. Our predecessors had ruled that it was wrong for naturally naked men to remain so. Wherever possible, they were urged and ordered to wear rags so that sheltered European minds might not be corrupted by the sight of human bodies. The natives, however, needed little urging.

The second reason they wore clothes was an extremely practical one—they helped to overcome the desert cold. We were also assured that clothes, even overcoats, helped to keep them cool on the hottest summer days by preventing the sun from making direct contact with the skin.

In spite of all this, we saw plenty of nakedness. Tribesmen brought in from the bush by the police for spearing cattle were invariably unclad.

Once a year the camels brought government-issue blankets and clothing for the natives. There were shirts for the men, frequently commandeered by the women, and rolls of cheap navy-blue serge which the government's housekeepers in Adelaide intended should be made into skirts...but by whom? The aboriginal women had never seen a needle and thread, and even if they had the skilled task of dressmaking would have been beyond their comprehension. Perhaps it was intended that each woman should cut off a length of serge, wrap it around herself, and tie it in place with a piece of grass-string. In any case, my mother took pity on them as usual and came to the rescue with her own skill and a small hand-driven sewing machine she had brought from Adelaide to make clothes for her family. I wonder what the average mother of today would say if suddenly confronted with the task of making sixty skirts... six would be bad enough, but sixty seemed a monumental undertaking. Yet that is the number she made; I remember clearly that the bolt of serge was measured and cut into that number of skirt lengths. The housegirls took turns to kneel by the little handmachine and wind frantically to my mother's instructions..."quick-time now!"..."all right, slow-feller."

The styles, mind you, weren't exactly what one might have expected in the latest batch of catalogues from the mail-order houses in Adelaide, Melbourne, and Sydney, and any self-respecting Parisian couturiere would have been horrified. The skirts were little more than serge sacks, hemmed at each end, one end having a tape which could be drawn into the wearer's waist. By this means, mother obviated the necessity for individual fittings. One size fitted all comers—from a teenage girl to a portly matron.

Telegraph station buggy outside Wallis's store, the township's leading emporium

This government wagon arrived at the station under 14 camel-power

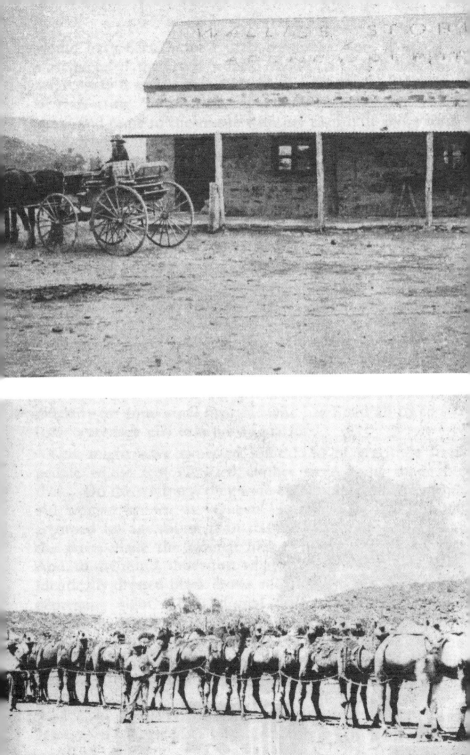

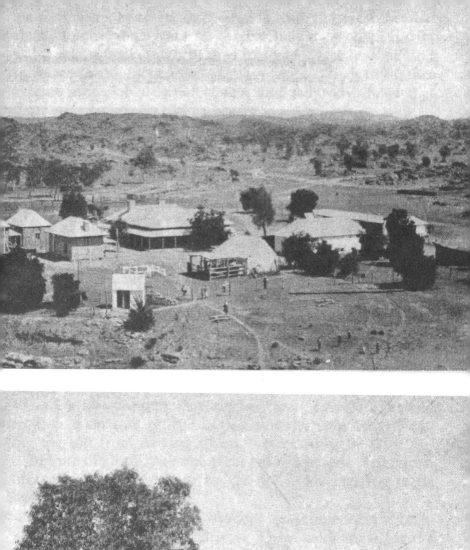

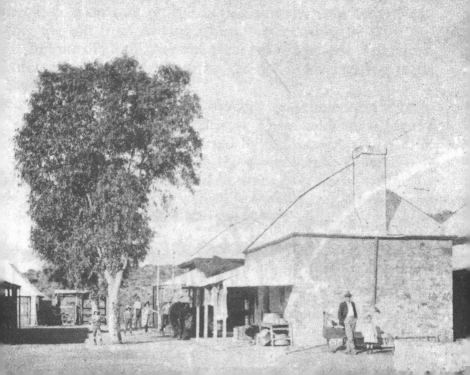

One might have expected some kind of gratitude from people whose first civilized clothes were being made for them. On the contrary, they were extremely ungrateful. One old woman known as "Queen" Luitchira—an honorific accorded for age rather than status—said disdainfully that the skirts made the women look "Allasame longa crows." And, to my mind, that's just what they did look like—sixty identically dressed black crows, moving in flocks, and a most depressing sight. This dismal aspect would have been relieved by a few bright plain colours, some reds and blues and yellows, but there it was—navy serge! No wonder the aborigines today like the strongest possible colours in their clothes. And how well they look in scarlet shirts and emerald green dresses. But there was nothing we could do about that in the early 1900s; we took the government-issue material and did our best with it; if the natives didn't like it they had to remain naked.

When my mother had finished the skirts there was a remnant of serge remaining. She tossed it to me and said, "There you are, Doris; you can make a pair of pants for Tommy Bungeye."

Poor Tommy was nobody's child, a twelve-year-old boy who had a mixture of Chinese and aboriginal blood in his veins, and therefore did not fully belong either to the aboriginal or the European world. His parentage was extremely obscure, especially on the paternal side; nobody seemed to know where he had really come from and few seemed to care. Although he lived in the aboriginal camp he was still something of an outcast among them and must often have felt totally depressed by this sense of not belonging to any group. In addition, he was cross-eyed and rather a sorry figure. I suppose I had

Two views of the telegraph station in 1907. It was then a bigger place than the township

previously expressed pity for him and now I had to justify it by making him a pair of pants. Tommy was delighted, waved the pants aloft, and ran around the station calling out, "Look, look, drawers!" At least he was the only one who received the handout with any show of enthusiasm or gratitude.

Every day the housegirls returned to their camp for an afternoon rest. It was a strict rule that before leaving they must change their house clothes. My mother knew that if they were taken to the camp they would be filthy within a few hours if they weren't given or gambled away. These clothes were undoubtedly the most fashionable worn by any of the aboriginal women on the station—a tidy uniform of bright print skirt worn over a man's shirt buttoned at the neck and the wrists. Over the shirt they wore a bandolier of red and brown bean seeds and a white band around the forehead to keep their hair in place. Some of them, especially a comparatively pretty girl named Amelia, might not have been out of place in a Rajah's palace. But teaching them elementary hygiene was difficult. They did not understand the necessity to wash. All their lives they had done without it, and couldn't see why they should bother about it now. Their siesta was spent in the dust of bush wurlies in the company of dozens of dogs and tribespeople who indeed never did wash. They lay on the ground around their campfires and frequently rolled into them. Campfire burns were a daily occurrence, but these injuries seemed to concern them less than others. In any case, when they returned to the house before the evening meal they wore unmistakable signs of where they had been; my mother had to be constantly on the alert to see that they washed before changing back into the uniform.

"Runge," she'd ask, "have you washed?" Runge was a dear old soul who was with us for years.

"Yes, Quei."

"Runge! True-feller? I smell plenty smoke on you."

Really on her dignity now, Runge would become expansive: "True-feller, Quei. Me bin have big-feller swim."

To an aboriginal whose environment had always been the arid desert, a wash in an enamel dish might have represented a big-feller swim, but it wasn't good enough for my mother. She realized that in order to keep disease away from us she must insist on their washing properly; if she wasn't satisfied that had been done she supervised a second dip, so to speak.

The evening meal and the washing-up had to be finished early each day so that the housegirls could get back to their camp before dark. Nothing would have induced them to be out alone, or even in company, once the light had gone—for it was then that the malevolent Kadaitcha Man stalked abroad. The Kadaitcha was an unseen devil with supernatural powers; he was the tribal bogy man, the tribal executioner (unexplained deaths were normally attributed to him) , and generally the terror of the neighbourhood.

The Kadaitcha Man really takes his name from shoes made of emu feathers, marsupial fur, and sacred blood taken from men's arms. I was overcome with revulsion the first time I saw a pair of these shoes and realized that they'd probably been worn by a tribal murderer or, more correctly perhaps, an executioner appointed by the elders. The Kadaitcha Man who wore the shoes had his little toes treated with hot stones and dislocated before putting them on. The broken toes were said to act as eyes to prevent a man intent on a stealthy killing from tripping on stones or twigs and thus betraying his presence. It was probably the cause of the widespread belief that a Kadaitcha Man could move without making any sound whatever. He was not inherently malevolent; in all cases he was said to have been sworn to his duty by others and to have refused to kill would have meant his own death. It wasn't surprising, therefore, that the housegirls insisted on being safely in their camps before the curtains of darkness fell; nor was I surprised to find that very few aboriginal men walked around at night except for the most pressing reasons.

Before long, the skirts my mother made were reduced to rags, and dirty ones at that. Many were converted into "headache" bands known as chilaras and were worn as such by men, women, and children. It amused us to see our dress materials bound around the heads of bearded men, but I'm not sure that it amused my mother quite as much; she had worked for hours to make the skirts and didn't appreciate their destruction. Headache bands, really a form of ornamentation, are still worn by the tribespeople today, but they use aspirins instead of bands to drive away aches. When we were there the Aranda believed that a headache could be squeezed out if the band was tied tightly around the forehead; it probably had the opposite effect of limiting circulation and aggravating the trouble. Poor old Runge had the greatest difficulty in keeping her chilara; inevitably it was taken from her by her selfish husband, a spoilt, only son, who regarded her as nothing more than a chattel.

The aborigines made their own chilaras with string woven from human hair, red ochre, and wax. Some were quite bright and bound in numerous layers around their heads; the band was sometimes three or four inches wide. Women's long hair was in heavy demand—even mine! At one time I had it growing half-way down my back. Old Jimmy, the current water-carrier, saw me drying it in the sun. He dropped his buckets, his mouth fell open, and he stared at it ecstatically.

"Good-feller string, Doriseel" he said. "You gib me?"

After my indignant refusal he laughed delightedly and went on his way. Thereafter we frequently play-acted this little pleasantry. Every time he saw me he'd go through the actions of rolling string, rubbing his hands down his skinny old legs, his eyes dancing with fun.

Alice Springs at the turn of the century wasn't exactly a mecca for touring concert parties which were then the rage in the south. Of course, we never saw one; the cost of travel and the tiny population made it economically impossible. So we had to make our own fun which, as I've already explained, often consisted of sing-songs in our home. But don't let it be thought that we didn't have concerts; on the contrary, they were there for the asking almost every night—in the natives' camp. Their corroborees seemed to be endless. Chanting and. the clack of beating sticks were so much a part of the background noises that, as with the song of birds, we soon became immune and unconscious of them. However, there were times when, strictly by invitation, we visited the camp and enjoyed these primitive concerts performed in the dust.

On one occasion Runge, the housegirl, begged Mother to go to the camp that night to watch a women's corroboree. But mother had been subjected to an earlier embarrassing experience and she wasn't keen to repeat it. She had gone with the current governess, Miss Mabel Taylor, and one of the operators, Leslie Spicer, and been shocked on arrival to find that all the women were completely naked.

"No, Runge," she said firmly. "That other time I go you give me big-feller shame—all those girls with nothing clothes..."

Runge obviously remembered that episode and was sorry for it. But she was terribly anxious that we should see them dance this particular corroboree.

"You come tonight, Quei, me tell'im allabout must wear shirt. True-feller."

My mother could see that she was sincerely crestfallen by the refusal, and eventually relented.

"All right," she said. "Suppos'im you promise to wear shirts we'll come tonight."

So mother, Miss Taylor, and I, escorted by Leslie Spicer, appeared at the appointed time in the vice-regal box—or, I should say, we sat on an empty box—and waited for the curtain to rise and the performance to begin.

The natives, as usual, were in no hurry. Time was the least of their worries. The advertised start was "after sundown." That could be interpreted as seven o'clock or nine o'clock as the mood suited them. They had no early doors, no last trains to catch, and no thought of tomorrow's work. They would begin when they were good and ready and not before. Eventually we learnt to walk to the camp when it was apparent from the warming-up of the "orchestra"—the Songman clearing his throat and a few tentative noises from the beating sticks—that the concert was about to start.

On this occasion the orchestra had taken its position in the pit. The men were clapping their hands, the sticks were beating, and a Songman was giving forth in a high-pitched multisyllabic voice. Then the performers appeared—the ladies of the ballet, so to speak—and began shuffling and stamping in long lines, the dust rising in clouds around them as their feet grooved into the soft red earth. They danced expertly and well, as the natives always did, but it could just as easily have been a strip-tease show in a low Parisian dive. From the front the women all appeared to be as Nature made them; there had been no attempt at concealment of any kind; and yet, true to Runge's promise, they did wear shirts—the sleeves tied around their necks and the rest flapping down their backs.

Runge arrived for work next morning bursting with pleasant anticipation of Quei's praise. What she heard instead was querulous disapproval.

"Oh, Runge, me properly big-feller shame!" my mother said.

Runge was dismayed but totally perplexed by this atti-tude. She did not speak, but her face was eloquent. It clearly said, "How is it possible to please white people? You asked us to wear shirts and we wore them and now you say you're ashamed. What must we do to win your approval?"

These corroborees were not our only form of entertainment. We also had the fun of watching wars. Yes, wars.

Real wars in which people were maimed and sometimes killed. But unlike the modern variety the lives of non-combatants were not in danger. Spear-bombs were not dropped on defenceless women and children; rather, like the emperors and senators of ancient Rome, we were given grandstand seats in a vast natural amphitheatre; from these vantage points we could watch unmolested as the shots were called and fired. If necessary, I'm sure they'd have waited for our arrival before beginning.

Runge and the other housegirls arrived for work one morning bubbling with the news that a war was imminent. There had been a breach of tribal protocol; either that, or some local Pearl Harbour had been attacked. In any case, Runge told us that a "properly big-feller mob" of foreign natives (they might have been from twenty or thirty miles away) were coming to fight the station tribesmen. Instead of asking for the evacuation of all women and children, as might be expected today, they hurried through the housework in order not to miss a moment of the approaching battle. Surprisingly, I was allowed to skip school for the rest of the day and go with my young brother, Mort, to watch the fray. He was then about seven and this was his first taste of war. Seventeen years later, at the age of 24, he was killed in France in a rather less civilized battle at Bullecourt.

We followed the women across the river to the Alice Springs Colosseum—a line of low hills which gave us a perfect view of the valley below. This was to be the battleground where the gladiators would meet and attempt to rend each other apart, or so I supposed. Actually, it didn't turn out quite that way.

A number of women were already in the stands. They were strangers who had come with the opposition, and we might have been expected to jeer them. There was a tense air of expectancy, that eve-of-Waterloo atmosphere preceding even the most modest drama. Eventually the combatants appeared, an equal number to each side which I thought was jolly sporting of them. They had obviously not heard of the sophisticated ideal of European generals who attempted to make war as unequal as possible by sheer weight of superior numbers. That would never have done for the Central Australian aborigines. "Not fair, not properly-way," they'd have said, and meant it.

At first I didn't recognize Our Side—the one I was to barrack for. They had thrown off the filthy old rags I had become accustomed to and were entirely naked; but their bodies were painted elaborately with red and white ochre and decorated with emu feathers, each according to the man's totem. They all carried spears and shields and, like the youths of today who anticipate the celluloid murders of television's Wild West, I suppose I looked forward to a gory battle. But in that I was disappointed; there was a most unsatisfying anticlimax.

The legions advanced in line abreast towards one another, brandishing their spears and yelling imprecations which would probably have been blood-curdling enough if I'd understood the language. I waited tensely for the spears to be thrown and for transfixed men to fall and groan. I realize now that if there had been any such likelihood I'd almost certainly have been kept well away. I became engrossed by a very aggressive young man—one of the visiting "baddies"—who was dressed in a hair-belt with a bunch of long emu feathers fastened to it. These bobbed up and down over his rear as he strutted boastfully and shouted what must have been dire insults at one of our station "goodies" named Bob. To my intense delight, Bob charged this pretentious braggart with his spear and I thought would have run him through; but the invader turned and ran like the emu he'd stripped, his arms flailing as he kept just a spear's length ahead. Oh, what delicious excitement this was for our lubras who screamed their pleasure, especially when every few yards Bob lunged with his spear and nipped off one of the fleeing feathers. I cheered him, too, but still had time to be aware of a visiting woman beside me who was apparently the Emu Boy's mother; she wailed piteously, a cry which was later translated to me as "Oh, my poor boy, my poor boy!" And poor boy he was; when I last caught a glimpse of him through the milling crowd there were only one or two bedraggled tail feathers left, and good old Bob looked like depriving him of those, too. He had been well and truly plucked.

As for spears being thrown in anger—well, that just didn't happen, although I was assured that it often did. This battle was rather more of a grievance settling than a full-scale war, a local border incident as we'd say today. I'm told there would have been a token letting of blood and thereafter all wrongs would be considered redressed. The discharge of steam did them all good; it made a conversation piece for weeks afterwards, especially the hilarious episode of Bob de-feathering the Emu, and nobody was seriously hurt. The intruders vanished as quickly as they came, and the inter-tribal relationships were then said to have been restored. Diplomatic exchanges were resumed—in the Aranda-pidgin phrase, all was said to be "level-feller." And I wouldn't be surprised if the visitors returned to our camp that night, by invitation, for a little conviviality and share-and-share-alike.

Chapter Six

PICNICS AND PICCANINNIES

MY MOTHER'S PATIENCE MUST HAVE BEEN seriously taxed by the long line of inept recruits to the position of housegirl. Some stayed for only a few weeks or a few months before going on their inevitable walkabouts, and mother then had to go through it all again..."No; that's not the way to wash dishes".."I want the floor swept—not half of it"... "No, the copper stick is not for burning; it's to get the clothes out"...teaching each one separately what she'd already been through a dozen times. The women seemed totally incapable of teaching one another, at least to my mother's standards of efficiency, so she had to do it herself. I must say that generally she retained her temper and her equanimity; but there was a limit and her name was Katie.

During one of the frequent staff shortages, Katie was hauled before my mother by her husband as a hopeful aspirant for the position of housegirl. Her qualifications for the job were nil; on the contrary, she started from well behind scratch because she had never been inside any kind of house in her life. She therefore had to be taught not only the work to be done, but the very walls and cupboards had to be explained to her. Katie was coy and an incurable giggler whose bouts of inane laughter became maddening after the first hour or so. She couldn't have been more than fifteen, but was well and truly "married" in the tribal fashion to a middle-aged man who already had another wife and family. There was nothing unusual about that, for the Aranda were traditional polygamists, but it was surprising that a husband should be trying to get rid of such a young woman as someone else's servant. Mother was reluctant to take her; she wanted a woman who at least knew the names of the rooms in a house and wouldn't enter the kitchen when told to fetch an article from the bedroom. However, the husband was so keen to get rid of Katie that he literally pushed her inside and, as far as he was concerned, she was then employed. In more sophisticated circumstances he would have made an excellent salesman.

Our first experience of Katie's capabilities, or lack of them, occurred on her very first day of duty. While we were at dinner the baby of the family cried in his cot. Mother called to Katie, "Bring'em baby alonga me," and waited hopefully for results.

Time passed and the baby continued to wail, but we thought Katie must be making progress by the sounds of bumping and thumping, grunts and giggles on the veranda. Eventually Katie appeared tugging a large cast-iron boiler across the floor. She had never heard of a baby. To her they were all piccaninnies. Apparently the only item she could think of beginning with "b" was the boiler.

That would have been laughed off if it hadn't been for Katie's discovery of scissors and what they were made for. She'd had a few delightful days exploring the house, poking into cupboards and drawers which she had no right to open. She had no idea, of course, that other people's privacy should be respected; there was no difference in her mind between opening the door of a room and the door of a cupboard. So that when she discovered that scissors were a cutting tool she immediately put them to use. Unfortunately she chose to try them on new curtains and a good tablecloth, giving them a fringe in places where fringes weren't intended. The damage was bad enough in itself, but worse still at Alice Springs because the curtains and the cloth would have to be replaced from Adelaide—and the camels weren't due just then. In these circumstances, I wasn't surprised that my mother rather uncharacteristically boiled over.

"Back you go! Back you go at once!" she said, insistent that she should leave the house instantly.

Poor Katie had to return crestfallen to her lord and master in the camp, where she would almost certainly have been given a good thrashing.

Fortunately they weren't all like Katie; her opposite was Runge, who stayed with us for years and was as efficient and loyal as others were silly and unreliable.

When mother was not feeling well Runge would put her arms around her protectively and say, "You go longa bed, Quei; me shepherd'em piccaninnies." And shepherd us she did, with all the gentleness and affection of one of our own relatives.

Shortly after the first World War, long after we had returned to Adelaide, Runge was one of the victims of a pneumonic influenza epidemic which swept through Central Australia. Hundreds died without medical aid, and dear old Runge was one of them.

When she knew she was dying Runge sent for my uncle, Ernest Allchurch, who was then in charge of the Alice Springs station.

"You tell'im Quei me go alonga Jesus," she instructed him.

That was a heart-warming message for my mother, who for years had gathered the lubras together every Sunday morning for simple religious instruction with large coloured pictures illustrating Bible stories.

I remember that one of these pictures, of Elijah being fed by the ravens, made a deep impression on a station lubra named Polly.

Later, when she gave birth to a son, Polly brought the baby

to mother to be given a "whitefeller" name. It was accepted custom for mother to name the aboriginal children, although, of course, they had their own tribal names. After several years of this, however, mother's supply of names was running low and she couldn't think of a new one.

Finally she said to Polly, "Well, I don't know, Polly, what name can we give him?"

"Tink'it 'Lijah good-feller name, Quei?" she said hopefully.

"Elijah! That's a Biblical name. Why do you want that name?"

Polly knew exactly why she wanted her son to be called Elijah. "Spose'im sit-down longa bush and got nothing tucker, God send'im tucker longa crows if call'im name 'Lijah."

So Elijah he was, and he grew into a fine man. He was one of the few Central Australian aborigines who enlisted in the army in the first World War.

Our horse-riding days were not without minor tragedies. The first of these occurred when I was learning to ride on a quiet old mare soon after we arrived. One day I ignominiously fell off, or was thrown off, and cut my ankle badly on a sharp flint. Subsequently it was balm to my wounded pride to learn that the accident happened because a stirrup strap broke; but that didn't help the injured flesh, especially when my father, in his inexperience, drenched it liberally with arnica, which was for use only on unbroken skin. That was roughly equivalent to pouring in salt, although at the time I thought that nothing could have been worse than the arnica, a tincture of wild tobacco, which scarified me like red-hot needles. My yells ran through the station and must have penetrated the native camp and even the township. Thereafter, my father apparently unwilling to face his daughter's screams, the duty of dressing my wound fell to the senior operator, Jim Field. I was pleased to know that he'd had more experience than my father at bush aid, and the arnica was replaced by iodoform, a more soothing powder.

I was laid up for a long time, but as soon as I was well enough I was in the saddle again, riding out through the hills with our scarlet-coated escort. Oh yes, we had an aboriginal escort in a scarlet coat. He looked almost as impressive as the Master of a Hunt Club, or the Clerk of the Course at Ascot. It's difficult to believe now, but postmen in Adelaide once wore a uniform of scarlet coats finished with brass buttons. When these were discarded for something more practical, an inspired official had them all sent to the Overland Telegraph stations for use by the native employees. Our grooms were the natural inheritors. For a time we really cut a dash as we rode through the small township escorted by a resplendent aboriginal in scarlet coat, turned-up hat, riding breeches, and leggings. Nothing like it had been seen in Central Australia. When we first rode down the Todd and along the street towards Heavitree Gap the mouths of those residents who saw us dropped open in surprise almost as though a company of the Horse Guards had suddenly been transported from Whitehall. But, as we might have expected with the aborigines, in no time at all Charlie the groom arrived for duty one morning dressed in his old shirt and trousers and looking more like a disreputable tramp than an elegant equerry.

When we asked what had happened to the uniform he replied unashamedly, "Paddy bin win'im longa euchre."

"Oh, did he!" my father exploded. "Well, you just go and win him back again. I don't care how—but you see you get that uniform."

That was more easily said than done. The complete ensemble had disappeared as if by magic and we never saw any of it again. Either Charlie was a better loser than a winner, in which case it's surprising that he didn't lose his own shirt and trousers too, or the uniform had been passed to another camp and perhaps even to another tribe for trade goods. Charlie returned to face the music and was soundly berated by my father, but at least we couldn't say that he hadn't tried to improve his appearance. During his absence he had washed his own clothes and returned wearing them—dripping wet.

It seems incredible now that natives who'd had only spasmodic contact with Europeans for thirty years should have so quickly acquired the white man's instinct for gambling. None of them could count beyond five, and yet they said they played euchre which involved the ability to add and subtract and to recognize the value of cards being played into a ring. This always puzzled us. I think they must have used the name euchre because they had heard it at the station in relation to cards; they probably played a much less complex game in which counting may not have been important. Whether that was so or not, there is no doubt that they were incurable gamblers. As they had no money they exchanged trade goods, food, clothes, and even wives. In time we got used to seeing treasured finery, which had been given to men and women for services rendered, being worn by various lucky winners; in fact, it seemed inevitable that clothes we gave away could never remain in the possession of the recipient. That being so it often seemed futile to make such presents.

Throughout our stay in Alice Springs we had to make our own fun. The beach was a thousand miles away. Radios and motor cars were still things of the future. We had no theatre, no church, no milk bar, no dance hall—none of those amenities which provide diversions for today's youth. We were cast upon our own resources and we made the most of it. School hours were shortened on Wednesdays so that we could go for a ride through the hills or along the river; Saturdays were often set aside for the special treat of a bush picnic. Nowadays people rush off to the hills at fifty miles an hour, stop at a roadhouse for a meal, and rush back again. They might travel two hundred miles or more in a day but seem to see little apart from the black-tarred roads most of them stick to. They come home suffering from nervous strain and probably frightened by near-misses which could have been bad accidents. Our picnics were really worthy of the name; they were restful and delightful and we returned tired but refreshed. We had time to explore, to prospect for minerals if we felt like it, or simply to lie in the warm sun until we were toasted or went to sleep. There was never any hurry. We went on picnics as though we were going out to enjoy ourselves, and we invariably did. My mother prepared hampers which made feasts of our picnic lunches—with a proper tablecloth laid out on the sand and food in bottles and jars and bags, and smoky billy tea with delicious scones. Well, yes, the flies were bad at times but we kept them at bay with gumtip switches. Often three or four families went out together on combined picnics, a most civilized form of social intercourse which regrettably appears to have passed from the lexicon of fun.

In spite of that it's a wonder our very first communal picnic, soon after we settled down, didn't discourage us forever. I'll never forget it. We had one to Emily Gap in the MacDonnell Ranges in two buggies. Mrs Charles Brookes, wife of the police constable, drove from their camp at Heavitree Gap with her four children and an aboriginal horseboy. On the way through Alice Springs she picked up Mrs Charles Meyers, wife of the saddler, and her two children. We contributed seven: my mother, the governess, four children, and Jack Supple, one of the operators, who drove us in the station buggy. What a day he must have had, with four women and ten children on his hands! However, I've always believed that telegraph operators were a longsuffering lot; he came along uncomplainingly and submitted to the kind of torture that grown men can expect from children.

We had an extremely pleasant day in the shadow of the ranges, searching for lizards when the mood was upon us, but most of the time we lazed and ate. The trouble began after the aboriginal harnessed the horses for the return trip and we were ready to move. At that moment the fractious police camp horses decided that home was never like this and that Emily Gap would do them. This was unusual behaviour. Horses are notoriously anxious to get back to their home pastures from any excursion, but this was certainly an exception. They were coaxed and whacked and dragged but they stubbornly refused to budge, perhaps having sensed that the only white man with us was not an experienced bushman. The buggy was dangerously near some washed-out gutters, dusk was falling, and the road home was a rough bushy track which certainly needed to be negotiated in daylight.

Mrs Brookes was an excitable woman and we thought she might become hysterical. On the contrary, she declared dramatically that she and the children would camp where they were for the night. As she had lived in the Centre longer than any of us we did not argue. In any case, it seemed the only sensible thing to do, although when we were safe at home and sitting around a fire I thought of her out there alone with the children in a land where wild aborigines still wandered. All the left-over picnic food, dried-out by exposure to the air, was thrust upon the Brookes, as were all our rugs and coats and anything else that might help them through the cold night. The rest of us, a total of ten when the Meyers family was included, somehow piled into our buggy and away we went, leaving the forlorn Brookes family to spend a lonely night. Since the advent of the internal combustion engine it has always been a reasonable excuse for delay to say that the motor broke down. But how was it possible to explain that the horses broke down? Did they run out of fuel? Not a bit of it; rather were they determined to stay around a good bowser. They weren't bogged, and they didn't have a flat tyre. All that could be said was that the horsepower had failed.

Darkness had fallen before we saw dim lights. Hundreds of natives' dogs yelped at the unseemly intrusion as we drove through the camp, and their owners, rudely awakened, gave us a long harangue on what they thought of people who travelled at night. Fortunately we didn't understand Aranda, and what I feel sure was abuse was lost on us. But it wasn't lost on the sensitive horses, which shied and became skittish and gave Mr Supple some trouble. The poor man must have anticipated being rid of us; however, he had another act of gallantry to perform before he could be let off the leash. Mrs Meyers had to be driven home. And on the way she remembered that before leaving that morning she had seen a snake slither into her bedroom. Her husband was away at Haasts Bluff...and would Mr Supple mind having a look...He looked while we watched from a safe distance; there was no snake in the bedroom and prodding with a stick produced nothing from a near-by hole. So Mrs Meyers had to be left alone with her babies with the knowledge that a live snake was some-where in the vicinity... but that was part of the price all women paid when they came to the outback. The thought of snakes couldn't have worried her too much though; after taking her children south to be educated Annie Meyers returned to Alice Springs and ran a boarding house for many years. In the days when food lacked variety and was often hard to get at all, running a boarding house for hungry men might have been a haunting experience worse even than the threat of snakes.

Next morning a rescue party, which included several good horsemen, went to Emily Gap to help Mrs Brookes. They found that she had spent most of the night rigging shelters over her children to prevent their being moonstruck. This was a derangement of the mind which, according to a widespread belief of the times, was caused by excessive exposure to the moon. She believed it and, what's more, so did I. From that time on I always rigged a parasol over me when sleeping in the open. The horses behaved like lambs when harnessed once more, apparently recognizing the voice of authority among our expert teamsters. After what must have been a terrible night for her, Mrs Brookes was delivered to the police camp. I don't remember her ever coming on another picnic and I can't say that I blamed her.

Like Mrs Meyers, she must have been terrified that she or her children would be bitten by snakes while sleeping on the ground. We saw them frequently at the telegraph station, generally on the veranda of the office. I remember the operators saying they believed the snakes were attracted by the ticking of the instruments. One of the operators, Phillip Squire, was a little disconcerted one night to find a snake coiled on the back of his chair and curiously looking over his shoulder. Perhaps they could read Morse code and were interested in the world news streaming through.

In later years Mrs Brookes developed serious eye trouble, as did many of the people who went to Central Australia. The aborigines suffered badly from trachoma, an infectious eye disease like an advanced form of sandy blight. After my father had consulted specialists in Adelaide by telegraph, Mrs Brookes was persuaded to go away for treatment. Mrs Meyers took the two youngest children to live with her, and mother brought the two eldest to the station to live with us. They also shared our school lessons—the first they'd ever had. Mrs Brookes was responding to treatment in Adelaide when she heard that there were several cases of typhoid fever at Alice Springs. This must have worried her to distraction, especially as she wasn't able to speak to her children and be reassured by them. All we could do was send telegrams to say they were all right. Nevertheless, she caught the next fortnightly train to Oodnadatta and came home on the mail buggy. Poor woman, she paid dearly for her foolish impulse. She soon had to return to Adelaide for further treatment and eventually lost her sight.

In the early years, Mrs Meyers was my mother's closest woman friend. Just how close that relationship was can be gauged from the fact that they helped one another through various confinements in a land where the nearest doctor was more than three hundred miles away. John Flynn's Australian Inland Mission reached the Centre only after we had returned to Adelaide. My mother gave birth to three children while we were at the telegraph station, and each time she was assisted only by Mrs Meyers. This saved the eighty-mile drive to Hermannsburg Mission, as Mrs Meyers had done for her earlier confinements. But it is not difficult to imagine the mental stress these women were subjected to in the knowledge that if complications occurred skilled medical aid would be out of reach.

As the Bradshaw numbers increased—there were eventually four boys and three girls at Alice Springs—the station buggy was found to be too small to accommodate us all. My father bought quite an historic one to replace it. An early governor of South Australia, Lord Kintore, had driven overland from Port Darwin to Adelaide in 1891. The buggy he used was brought back to Central Australia in 1901 by Professor Sir Baldwin Spencer and Mr F. J. Gillen during their second expedition among the aboriginal tribes, and when they had done with it my father took it over from them. If still in existence the old buggy would be a museum piece; it was so heavy that five horses instead of the usual four were needed to draw it and the load of Bradshaws.

Simpson's Gap, about' fifteen miles from the telegraph station, was the farthest limit for a day's picnic, and even then it had to be saved for special occasions. Thirty miles in a day with a full load was as much as the horses could manage. Although I've never been back to Alice Springs, I'm told that Simpson's Gap can be reached today in twenty minutes. I feel sure the people who go there in that time don't have half the fun we had. The dry bed of the Todd, with its shady river gums and lovely ghost gums, provided wonderful picnic spots almost anywhere along its length. Our favourite was Wigley Waterhole, a few miles north of the station; it was not only a most picturesque place but had the novelty of water as well. Only those people who have lived in a vast arid region for any time will appreciate how we felt about being able to splash in a waterhole occasionally. Our dried-out spirits were resurrected by the very sight of it, and lathering our bodies and washing away the dust amounted to what was little less than a religious rite.

Imagine how we reacted, therefore, when storm clouds infrequently formed over the Centre and the skies poured forth enough water for the Todd and Charles rivers to cascade through the hills. Unfortunately, the flow seldom lasted more than about twenty-four hours; after that a few rockholes would remain filled but the rest of the water soon disappeared into the thirsty sand. That happened at the Wigley, too. My diary for 6th January, 1906, reminds me:

> "Started for the Wigley about 3 o'clock. Mort, Consie, and I rode, while others came in the buggy. Hardly any water there. But on the way back we saw two snakes." [As though *that* was compensation.]
>
> "January 8: Started school this morning. Temperature 107 degrees."
>
> " January 23: Only 112 degrees today." [I can't remember why I included the "only" in that entry unless the previous few days had been hotter still.]

My diary seems to have been largely preoccupied with a discussion of the weather, as if that would interest posterity. However, it has been a pleasant experience to read again my youthful reactions to the winter cold and the roaring log fires, to the storms we were caught in while riding, and to the apparently interminable picnics.

> "August 23: Went for a little picnic at the wood near Stuart Claypans in the township. [Now East Side, Alice Springs.] As soon as this was decided we had to let Mrs

Meyers know, of course, so we sent her a paper-yabber wedged in a cleft stick and carried by a black boy. He was fortified for his long walk with a stick of tobacco as pay and went away happily enough."

I remember that Mrs Meyers walked over and spent the day with us. We might all have been much more comfortable either at her home or at the telegraph station, where at least we would have had some refuge from the ants if not from the flies. But we enjoyed romping in the bush and the al fresco meals and, as I said, there were few other diversions. Despite Mr Stipple's experience, the men on the station were all very good-natured about our picnics; with the exception of the operator on duty they came with us frequently, riding ahead and behind like a Royal escort, but generally behind to save us from their dust. Three children, including myself, normally formed part of the mounted escort.

On "big" picnic days there was no more important man on the station than Harry Kunoth—and he knew it! His expert handling of the horse teams was a delight to watch. At an appointed hour Harry would arrive near the kitchen door in the new buggy hauled by its team of five. There mother superintended the packing of the tucker boxes into the tray of the buggy. Picnics always meant more work for her than for anyone else; she did all the baking and then prepared the food she had cooked; at the picnic site she laid it out and served it, then repacked what was left for the trip home—although I must say there were seldom any leftovers. She never allowed the aboriginal women to handle our food. The remoteness of medical aid made the possible transference of disease a paramount consideration, and the natives still had a long way to go in their understanding of hygiene. After the tucker boxes were aboard, the children, from four to seven of us, the governess, an aboriginal woman, and finally mother climbed up. Although she travelled thousands of miles in buggies during our nine years in Central Australia, she never became closely attached to the horses and couldn't distinguish any of them by sight. But she did know she disliked a skittish mare named Diana, a flighty show-off constantly hogging centre-stage with her antics. She was bad-tempered as well and could be thoroughly nasty.

Mother feared the worst each time Harry said, when it was her turn to board, "Get up quickly as you can Missus, and quietly," while never taking his eyes from two nervous aboriginal horseboys at Diana's head, trying vainly to anchor her to the ground.

"Now, Harry, you haven't got that Diana in the team again, have you?" she'd ask, never really knowing which one was Diana.

"Of course not, Missus," Harry would lie comfortingly. "Wouldn't think of it. You right now?" Then he'd tighten up the reins, give Diana a special flick to show her who was boss, and the picnic would be off to a flying start.

My father escaped the picnics as often as possible. He never could see any sense in them. He was a phlegmatic, studious man, who would rather spend his leisure with Dickens in England or Conrad on the high seas than be cast upon the mercy of flies, ants, and fretful children. However, it would never have done for us if he'd always stayed behind, so he came occasionally (if only to take a photo) and submitted with good grace to the torments that beset him.

One picnic at Simpson's Gap got this simple entry in his diary: "All station to Simpson's Gap picnic."

Just the bare statement of fact. No imagination, and certainly no enthusiasm —almost a "thank goodness that's over" attitude.

But my diary for the same date waxes positively lyrical:

"Mr Henry Fitz, the manager of Undoolya station, came in yesterday with the horse he promised I should ride to the Simpson's Gap picnic. Bluey is a grand horse! Mr Fitz wanted me to try riding in a man's saddle but I wouldn't [being a perfect lady at 15] so he put my side-saddle on him and I had a canter. Bluey is just lovely. We got a good start for the picnic. Mr O'Grady from the Arltunga goldfield was waiting in the township to join us. Bluey was pulling and wanting to race, but behaved when asked. He had been used to pace racehorses. It was lovely and we had such fun. In the evening, after we'd ridden home, everyone came to tea at the station, and afterwards we had a sing-song. Had a lovely evening."

I wonder how many fifteen-year-olds today would find such fun among a crowd of grown-up men and women? We always looked forward to Mr Fitz's visits; he was a gay, grey-moustached man with a rollicking Gaelic manner.

Mr Standish John O'Grady was manager of the battery at the Arltunga goldfield, about fifty miles away. Like Mark Twain, he once had the privilege of reading in the newspaper a report of his own death. The report, as Twain said of his, was grossly exaggerated. He died in Adelaide in 1963.

Arltunga was a flourishing goldfield before the turn of the century, but because it was more than a day's drive away we seldom went there, although I have vivid memories of the field. Gold from the mines—thousands of pounds worth—was sent in the buggy mail to Oodnadatta once a fortnight. And without an escort. It seemed like an open invitation for men cast in the same mould as the goldbushrangers of eastern Australia, and yet I never heard of a pennyweight being reported missing. One good reason, of course, was that anyone who robbed the coach was prevented by the desert from taking a route other than the single track that led into Oodnadatta or back to Alice Springs. Gold won't buy water in that country.

It was taken for granted after a special picnic for visiting men—our equivalent of today's barbecues and cocktail parties—that everyone would come back to the station for a sing-song; it was also taken for granted that anyone who could contribute would bring his music or his instrument and share in entertaining. Some of the men on the telegraph staff, and some at Arltunga, had fine trained voices, certainly the equal of most of the people who are called "well-known" singers on the present radio programmes. Nor did they find it necessary to sob, gyrate, gesticulate, or affect long hair-dos; what's more, the songs they sang are as imperishable now as then. One or two of the men were violinists, and the governess was always a pianist, as many women were in those days. Later I had to do my share as accompanist when I was sufficiently proficient. We had bought a piano from the Gillens on our arrival in 1899; that, like everything else, must have been carted in a horse-drawn wagon and sometimes it showed the signs of this long trip. Yet nobody was too critical, realizing that piano tuners were unknown in Alice Springs. One of the qualifications for all our governesses was that they must be able to play and teach the piano so, in turn, I was taught by Miss Bertha Easom, Miss Elsie Conigrave, Mrs Louisa Cornock, and Miss Mabel Taylor.

One of our favourite entertainers was Mr Fitz. He was the Bing Crosby of my youth and I never tired of listening to him. I always wheedled him into singing several parodies, including one sung to "In the Gloaming":

"On the ocean, oh my darling,
Cling not quite so close to me,
For I often at short warning
Wish to view the deep blue sea."

Then he'd lie back in his armchair, pipe in hand, and sing very softly,

"Oh bairnies, cuddle doon,"

with all the charm of his Irish-Scots ancestry. Perhaps he would launch into a recital of funny experiences which had befallen him, and funnier people he'd encountered; he'd enjoy the memory so much and laugh so heartily that he could gasp only a few words at a time; we would become infected by his hilarity and laugh with him until we were all quite hysterical.

How naive it all sounds now; but remember we had neither radio nor gramophone; we'd never heard a pop singer or even an honest old crooner like Bing Crosby; we certainly had no conception of what would be called "entertainment" half a century later.

Once we became amateur speleologists and explored caves at Temple Bar, south of the MacDonnell Ranges. Our leader in this expedition was Mr H. J. Hillier, an English teacher at Finke River Mission, Hermannsburg, and a wellknown naturalist. He was also an artist who did more than two thousand exquisite drawings of Central Australian insects and other specimens for the British Museum. Now he was looking for white bats—weird parchment-coloured creatures known to inhabit the caves.

The caves had never been explored. Rather than caves, they looked more like tunnels leading from a pit on the Emily Plain. Hillier thought they may have been an ancient creek bed which had subsided.

It was all terribly exciting. We crawled in on our hands and knees, and in very confined passages had to drop almost to our faces. Each of us carried a candle to test the air; we knew that if they sputtered and went out there would be insufficient oxygen to keep us alive. As we got farther into the dirty dark hole I looked forward more and more to the time when we would turn back for the exit. And how thankful I was that the bats were not at home; I had spent much of the time underground telling myself not to yell if one struck me. I was also relieved to emerge again into the sweet-smelling air—but not half as glad about it as an aboriginal horseboy who went with us but refused to enter the caves. As far as he was concerned, evil spirits dwelt there and he wanted no part of them. I'm sure he thought that we would all be gobbled up. While we were inside he took the horses well away from the entrance, not because of better grazing for the animals but because he wanted to put as much country as possible between himself and the entrance.

One afternoon we rode to Undoolya station to see Mr Fitz, only to find that he was away on a mustering trip with all his stockmen. But the cook, Charlie Towers, entertained us at afternoon tea in the kitchen. From there I could just see his small adjoining room, which to my fascination was lined from floor to ceiling with beautifully bound books. He was a tall, bearded man, one of those mysterious Englishmen who drifted to the outback—presumably as far as they could get from their homeland—and stayed there. My father knew more about Charlie Towers than any of us. As a special magistrate he had witnessed the signing of documents in which Charlie was said to have renounced his claim to a title and a large estate in England; but father was as maddeningly uncommunicative about Charlie's real identity as he was about the daily news of the world passing through the telegraph station. We never did find out. Nevertheless, I had seen enough to know that Charlie had the benefit of a superior education. That rough stone homestead at Undoolya must have been a humble place after the great halls he'd been used to. And one knew just by speaking to him that his rank was Gentleman as well as Camp Cook. The camel-freight on his books alone must have cost a small fortune.

Inspired by an article in an English children's magazine, I once organized a paper-chase on horseback. The two "foxes" led us through the township and Heavitree Gap to the vicinity of Mount Blatherskite, but the English author of the game hadn't reckoned on a hawk-eyed Australian bushman joining in. Harry Kunoth rode with us as one of the "hounds" and didn't bother to glance at the paper clues scattered by the "foxes" as they travelled. He rode at a hard gallop over rocky hills and through the scrub, simply following the tracks left by the leaders. We arrived at the finishing point almost simultaneously. When I thought of the hours I'd wasted tearing up paper it seemed a decided washout.

What fun we had, though, when dozens of wild donkeys were rounded up by the stockmen and brought in from the bush. Some of the men and two or three young Bradshaws managed to get on their backs, but I was fifteen, the dignified eldest member of the family, and I had to "know my place." Anyway, that was a good excuse for not trying to ride one myself. I was a little disconcerted by the pandemonium as the donkeys galloped around the station in all directions, almost colliding at corners, the riders yelling at each other as they tore past without hope of guiding the reinless animals.

During the short time they were kept on the station the donkeys grew quite docile. One of the stockmen made a small go-cart for the younger children; equipped with four wire and two wooden wheels which had been painstakingly fashioned. A donkey was then harnessed to the cart, the children piled aboard, and they were led around by an aboriginal. It became the family pram.

As my younger brothers and sisters grew older they each learnt to ride; they also learnt the art and the meaning of mischief. Modern youth has mischief tailor-made for him in the big cities; but in Alice Springs sixty years ago it had to be invented. Let me say that my brothers and sisters sometimes showed that they were inventive geniuses. Their childhood was ideally happy, and full of interest. But there had to be added spice to compensate for the drudgery and dullness of school lessons given by untrained teachers without any of the present-day aids. Perhaps that explains a plan I overheard being hatched by the younger children which was intended to discourage the newest governess from settling down, or at least from getting the impression that she was teaching a family of tame little angels. I felt it was time for intervention when they agreed that the governess should be greeted on the first day or so by being lassoed.

"And I'll tie her to a tree," one of the boys said.

"Yes, and while you're doing that I'll sool snakes on her," another said.

Of course, nothing of the kind was allowed to happen. Governesses, whether trained teachers or not, were far too precious to be made to feel that they should catch the first buggy back to Adelaide. One of them almost did when she discovered on her first evening that tea was invariably served at 5.30 p.m.

"It's not civilized to eat at such an unearthly hour," she complained.

But she had the choice of eating then with the rest of us, or getting her own meal later and doing her own washing up. The housegirls had to be back in the camp before dark; that was an inflexible requirement dictated by the nocturnal habits of the Kadaitcha Man, and in time even the governesses came to accept it. At 5.30 Cookie Lloyd hit an iron triangle with a bar. Nobody could possibly use the excuse that he or she hadn't heard the gong—it could be heard in the township two miles away.

The hours between tea and bedtime were the happiest of the day—a period of enchantment of the simplest kind that was our equivalent of the children's session and horse operas on television. Before darkness fell the men joined the children in a games session, whether cricket, rounders, throwing the ball, or foot-racing. Occasionally we had firecrackers, until one night when Harry Kunoth's pet foxterrier, Tike, caught a double-bunger in its mouth and held it there until it exploded. The dog was badly burnt, and for a long time thereafter was a very subdued animal.

At dark the younger children were sent to bed at once and I, even at sixteen, had to follow not a minute later than nine o'clock. In this respect I was strictly controlled by the governess and not by my parents. I'm sure she never knew how often I shook my fist at her as I went.

But between dark and the time when I had to leave there was generally an hour or two for yarning. The men invariably drifted over to our communal veranda from their own cramped quarters to enjoy the evening air and the comradeship of a handful of people with common interests who found themselves a thousand miles from their homes. Deck chairs were drawn close together, symbolizing the harmony of our self-contained community. Pipes were lit and the tranquil stillness was allowed to immerse us all for long periods before anyone spoke. And when someone at last broke the silence it might have been to talk of sealing wax, or cabbages, or kings—but most probably it was about the horses or the bullocks or the omnipresent O.T. Line. There might be stories of earlier days and strange experiences, of queer characters and queerer places. And I would sink deepdown into my deck-chair, remaining silent but absorbing all, as inconspicuous as I could be while dreading that detested "Time for bed, Doris!" The governesses, without consulting a watch, seemed to know clairvoyantly that in one minute the clock would strike nine. They gave me that much grace! Meanwhile, I enjoyed every moment.

A voice, low and unhurried and interrupted by puffs on a pipe, would come from the depths of a chair:

"You know...the best horseboy I ever had at Barrow Creek had a tail...an extra joint in his spine. Now that's a fact. It protruded so much that he couldn't ride a barebacked horse and we had to cut a hole in the seat of the saddle he used. But nothing on four legs could throw him..it seemed to anchor him there, and he did a marvellous job." The speaker may have been Jim Field or Leslie Spicer, both of whom served at Barrow

Creek, but you knew who spoke only by the tone of voice. The face was invisible except when occasionally illuminated by a match being applied to a cold pipe.

And from another chair: "Did I ever tell you about Charlie Brookes the policeman taking a tracker and another boy out to the western MacDonnells to search for six cattle killers?"

A question there, but nobody answered; it wasn't necessary; even if the story had been told a dozen times we could listen again.

"Well, when they got to the locality where the natives were hiding Charlie camped at a waterhole and, as usual, gave his trackers a rifle each and told them to go and bring in the killers. They returned the same afternoon. Charlie was surprised to see them so soon, but more surprised still to find they no longer had the rifles.

"'Which way those prisoners?' he asked.

"'Him come be'hind.'

"'Which way rifles?'

"'Bin leave'im longa those cattle killers; him bin want to shoot kangaroo.'

"Well, Charlie wasn't too happy at being left with nothing but his revolver. But at sunset the six boys came in, carrying two kangaroos and the rifles, and submitted quietly to being handcuffed and chained to a tree. They were each given six months in gaol at Port Augusta and had to walk to Oodnadatta; when they got there a mistake in their committal papers was discovered so they walked back to their own country. That was six hundred miles they walked in a few weeks. Think of that!"

I thought about it all right. I could think of nothing else, and before my eyes I saw again those pulped human feet I'd seen at Oodnadatta on the day we arrived.

Then there was another voice: "Out at Owen Springs station one time Spence Gall, the manager, caught a tenfoot snake—not venomous. Spence knew a zoologist was on the way from the south...a professor bloke...and he thought he'd be glad to have the specimen, so he kept it in a box on the veranda for a few weeks. Fed it on mice and all sorts of things. Well, when the professor came he had only packhorses and no means of carrying the snake alive, and he didn't have the right stuff to preserve its skin. So they let it out and watched it crawl over the creek to its lair. But apparently that snake had lost interest in the wide open spaces; next morning it was back in the box."

My father chuckled. It reminded him of a story, he said. "A chap from Hergott Springs told me about two men who were driving along in a cart..."

"Doris, it's time for bed."

"...and they saw a perentie, a giant goanna you know, and thought it would be fun to run over it. But the perentie had other ideas; it ran up and into the cart and the two men scrambled out in a panic..."

"Doris!..."

"...the old horse just kept jogging on, leaving them gazing after the perentie in full possession, sitting up on the seat with a slightly surprised look as it moved its head from side to side, wondering whether it should pick up the reins or not...oh, yes, goodnight Doris."

And as I walked to bed I was aware that the infrequent sounds from the natives' camp had ceased. The silence of the vast country had grown deeper. The stars were so brilliant and so apparently close that they seemed not countless but countable. Soon the little station in the, heart of Australia would be silent too, the only light in the office, the only sounds the soft incessant ticking of the Morse instruments, watched by the lone man on duty, and his steps every four hours as he went quietly across to the weather compound to take his observations and relay them to Adelaide.

Chapter Seven

DOCTOR
WHITEFELLOWS

IF EVER I FEEL NOSTALGIC ABOUT THE YEARS at Alice Springs I have only to open my own diary or my father's. Then at once I am transported back through half a century of time and a thousand miles of the outback to the tiny settlement that was my home for nine years—and although I haven't returned since we left in 1908 I can see it as clearly as if it all happened last week.

Hundreds of unimportant incidents that would otherwise have been forgotten are preserved for ever in these pages. I would never have remembered that a well-known geologist, Dr Charles Chewings, arrived in December 1902 to superintend operations at the Winnecke goldfield, or that my father opened a post office there in September 1903. Here again I see a note about the tremendous undertaking of carting the treatment plant to Winnecke from the Oodnadatta railhead. The smaller parts could be carried on camels after dismantling, but the huge boiler weighing several tons which was used to drive the machinery had to be brought in a wagon. On that trip Dr Chewings and his assistants were six weeks crossing the Finke River alone.

I might have forgotten the visit by the South Australian Government geologist, H. Y. L. Brown, who came on camels in

June 1902 for his regular inspection of mines in the Northern Territory. After visiting Arltunga and Winnecke he then left for Kurundi goldfield two hundred miles to the northwest.

I see that Professor Sir Baldwin Spencer and Mr F. J. Gillen were with us in April 1901. Mr Gillen had already collaborated with Professor Spencer on their book, *The Native Tribes of Central Australia,* and he had now been given a year's leave of absence from the P.M.G's Department for further field work among the aborigines.

There are notes on line inspections, the movement of sheep and horses to other telegraph stations, reports of court cases in which my father adjudicated, lists of stores, and the comings and goings of the surprisingly frequent travellers, all of them reminding me vividly of incidents that take me back easily to the day they happened. How well I remember the aboriginal stockboys leaving every few months with flocks of sheep for Barrow Creek, generally in response to telegrams that mutton farther north was becoming short. And how well I remember the arrival in March 1906 of a party of government geologists who had been on a prospecting trip to the Petermann Ranges in the far south-western corner of the Northern Territory. They were in a sorry state. They had encountered excessive summer heat (fancy going out there in summer anyway!) in a waterless area and underwent hardships such as have fallen to few.

As though that wasn't sufficient punishment, they were attacked while sleeping by wild Loritja tribesmen near the Ruined Rampart on 5th December 1905. One of the prospectors, T. W. Hall, was speared in the eye, and another, H. Fabian, in the chest. Their leader, F. R. George, nursed the wounded men under these terrible conditions until they were well enough to travel. They reached us on 29th March 1906. I know because my father's diary entry for that day says simply: "Mr George arrived." Three words to describe what was undoubtedly one of the epic journeys of the decade. And then there are two matter-of-fact entries for 4th April, just five days later:

"Mr George died 5 a.m.—dysentery."

"Mr George buried 4 p.m."

He had been worn out by anxiety for the safety of his men and the hardships they had undergone. He was a man of indomitable courage, and only thirty-two years old.

My father's diary was a small black book about four inches by three inches, but that and his medical diary contain the record of our times and have the power to transport me there again whenever I feel in the mood. Some of the laconic references to illnesses and injuries make me almost blanch when I remember the conditions under which they were treated; yet I marvel how my parents coped with each situation as it arose—a city office worker who had never had one lesson in first aid and a young housewife and mother who'd never been out of a suburban street.

Now take this for a typical piece of understatement, but also an indication of what had to be done in emergencies:

Oct. 21, 1901: Fitz, Dixon, DuBois and Schute capsized buggy driving in from Undoolya. Dixon's right thigh broken.

Oct. 22: Dixon's thigh set.

Nothing more than that. And yet behind it there is a remarkable story of fortitude and bush-aid.

Harry Dixon was one of the station operators who had been visiting Undoolya. How well I remember the ominous hush that fell over the station the morning his thigh was set. My father, of course, had spent much of the night in telegraphic consultation with a Doctor Marten who had been summoned to the G.P.O. in Adelaide to relay his instructions to Alice Springs. There they are in my father's neat handwriting in the medical diary:

"Place the patient on his back on a mattress with a board underneath to keep it level. Take a piece of wood two inches square, make a hole in the centre and put a cord through this. Take a strip of adhesive plaster two yards long by two inches wide and fix on both sides of the leg from just above the knee to the ankle, leaving undivided end as a loop below the foot. In the centre of the loop put the piece of wood with the cord coming away from the leg. Make a pulley and fix to foot of bed on a level with the foot, run cord over this pulley (a cotton reel with a piece of telegraph wire threaded through it) and apply 7 lb. weight to cord. Put a bandage around the plaster to keep it tight. Make long bags about as thick as the thigh to reach from the armpit to the foot on the injured side, and a bag to fit on the inside of the leg from the crutch to the foot, and fill them with sand. Also make a short bag to lie over the fracture transversely. Administer half a teaspoonful of solution of morphia in water. When done, and plaster fixed to leg, raise the foot of the bed six inches and get some strong men to hold the hips and lower part of the body while the "operator" and other strong men pull on the leg. [Oh, it's nothing; just a broken thigh!] They should pull directly against the men at the body. When the leg seems straight and nearly as possible the same length as the other, put it to lie on its back with the toes pointed directly upwards, and so place the sandbags as to keep the leg in a fixed position; then put the small bag directly across the line of the fracture. Keep him under the influence of morphia by administering in water every three or four hours or oftener if necessary. Patient will have to lie on

The Stuart Arms as we found it. Today it is an ornate five-star tourist resort

One of the first homes in Stuart village, later Alice Springs, belonged to Mr and Mrs Charles Meyers, seen with their family and staff

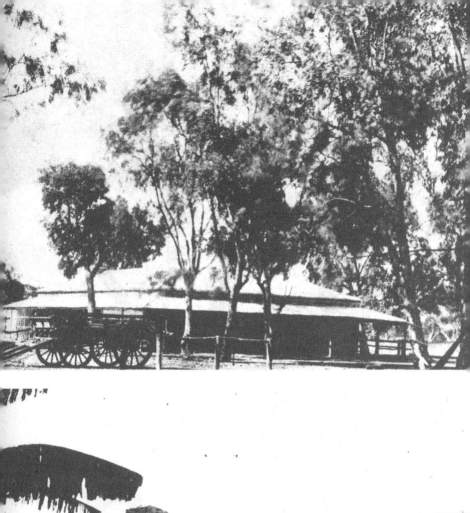
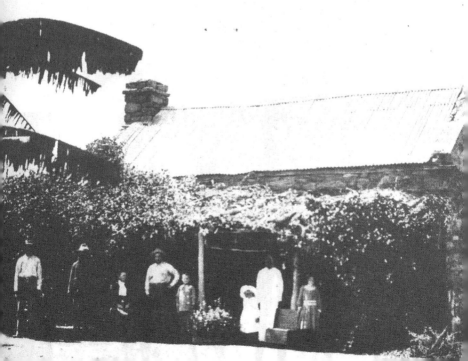

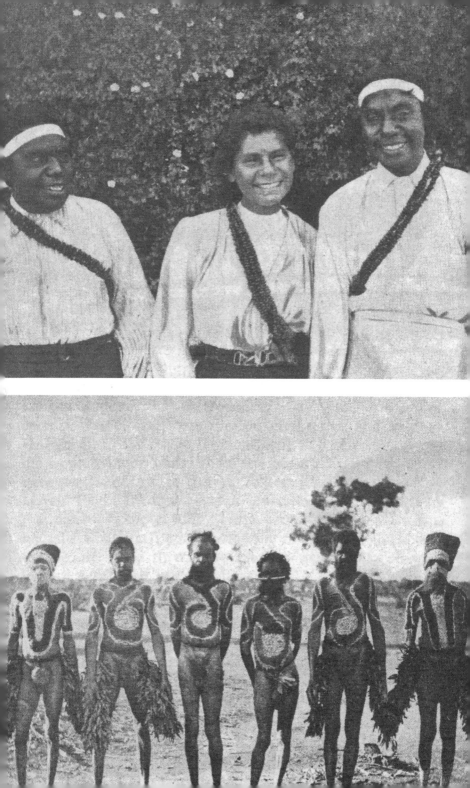

his back six or eight weeks. Apply spirits of wine to the back night and morning. Six weeks from accident take off all dressings, weight, etc., and move leg about a little. Then carry leg in a sling and use crutches, and gradually put weight of body on leg."

Well, that was all—and every word of it was received by my father in Morse code. He followed the instructions to the letter, except that I think he regarded the morphia as an anaesthetic and tried to render poor Mr Dixon unconscious with it. I know that he gave such massive doses to ease the pain while setting the leg that the patient complained of heart pains. This was referred again to Dr Marten, who prescribed a mustard plaster over the heart. The other operators took turn about to nurse him in their own quarters. They cared for him like a baby, made crutches for his convalescence, and assisted him to take his first hesitant steps after lying for weeks in his room in the summer heat. Mr Dixon recovered completely and in later years had only a very slight limp. My father must have taken that for granted because there is no subsequent reference to him in the diary. One would have thought that an amateur Doctor Whitefellow might have succumbed to the temptation of at least a two-word entry, "Dixon better." After such a triumph he might even have been pardoned for boasting a little: "Am glad to report that following my ministrations Harry Dixon's leg is mended, and he now walks again almost as liven, as ever." Not a bit of it!

There were other equally pressing problems. Father's brother, Ernest Bradshaw, a gentle courteous man of twenty-seven, had come from Melbourne to a drier climate which was thought might help a serious chest complaint. He got two words also.

Our house girls — Arnboora, Amelia, and Runge

Station aborigines dressed for a corroboree

July 18: Ernie arrived.

Six months later there were three entries.

Jan. 26: Ernie seized with coughing fit about midnight.

Jan. 28: Ernie died about midnight.

Jan. 29: Ernie buried 6 p.m.

Seven days later, on 5th February there was an almost verbose entry:

"32 camels with loading for Spencer and Gillen passed through to the north, and another ten loaded flour for them which has been lying at Alice Springs."

My Uncle Ernest was the third bookkeeper in succession to develop tuberculosis while employed by a Melbourne company. After his death, such were the beliefs and superstitions only sixty years ago, the management decided to destroy the books. Father had thought the Alice Springs climate would help him but hadn't realized how seriously ill he was; he should never have attempted the exhausting journey.

But the births outnumbered the deaths, at least among the Bradshaws. Three months before my uncle died my third brother was born. He was the first of three Bradshaw children born in Alice Springs, a fact which inspired a cousin in Adelaide to say, "Won't it be funny when Auntie brings home four white children and three black children."

Mrs Meyers, young and inexperienced, came to help mother, as mother went to her, later on, but I'm sure that mother's suffering in later years was traceable to the lack of proper medical care during our nine years in the Centre.

Perhaps the arrival of his fifth child missed my father's diary by accident or perhaps, already having four, he had become quite blase about it. In any case, the birth of Stuart MacDonnell Bradshaw (to commemorate his birthplace) was not recorded. To be sure, we learn that on 9th August 1900 "first lot of annual stores arrived." On 11th August "second lot of annual stores arrived." On 20th August "third ditto."

Mounted-Constable Brookes's departure with prisoners for Port Augusta was noted, as was a message from a man named Foster that one of his horses had knocked up about thirty miles from Alice Springs on a mail trip to Barrow Creek. But the arrival of Donnell, as we called him, escaped my father's notice altogether. Looking through the diary again I see that this was in keeping with his almost total lack of acknowledgment of our existence, except for illness and the sizes of our shoes. The diary, I assume, was for matters outside the family circle, for there are extremely few references to any of us. We broke into print once on 12th September 1904, when my mother took us all for a holiday in Adelaide.

"Mrs B. and family left for Oodnadatta."

Mort and I made the grade when we passed a drawing examination conducted by the Adelaide School of Design and I appeared there alone during a serious illness which must have worried him and my mother.

From the symptoms given by my father over the telegraph to the doctor, who was brought to the G.P.O. in Adelaide, it appeared that I had rheumatic fever. For a reason which was never understood—unless it was that he thought I had no chance—the doctor was uncharacteristically vague about treatment and nursing and my condition grew steadily worse. Mother wasn't cheered, and I'm sure I wouldn't have been either if I'd known, when some of the old hands remembered that the only other person who had contracted rheumatic fever in the Centre had died. He was Mr Ernest Flint, the station master who had gone to Alice Springs after escaping the attack by tribesmen at Barrow Creek in which Mr Stapleton and Mr Franks were speared to death. He and my Uncle Ernest Bradshaw were lying side by side in the little station cemetery and it seemed that I was to join them.

At last someone suggested trying to get in touch with the wife of a station-owner living near Katherine as she had been the matron of Port Darwin Hospital and might know something about medicine. Katherine was eight hundred miles away, but somehow she was contacted and gave practical advice which was recorded in my father's medical diary. I was to have hot baths, hot fomentations, warm clothing, my joints and limbs were to be bandaged in lint, and I was to be kept in bed, where I'd been for weeks (this in the middle of summer) : I was to be kept on a milk diet and take salicylic acid every four hours. It might not sound like the treatment a rheumatic fever patient would be given in a modern hospital today, but at least my torment of pain was relieved and I survived. To make matters worse, drought was upon the land and the stench of animal death was inescapable. As my condition improved I felt almost that I had been put out to starve with the melancholy cattle—a milk diet is not a proper ration for a growing girl. However, when I finally got out of bed and put on my clothes I found that I'd grown so much that some dresses wouldn't fit me.

Fortunately for us, our water supply wasn't affected by the frequent droughts. It was lovely water, filtered through the sand of the river bed and drawn from a soakage, the clear permanent waterhole below the station which gave to it its name. But other necessities were scarce so my mother had to use all her ingenuity to make meals palatable without butter, eggs, or fruit, and a drought-ration of milk and scarcely a vegetable. We didn't even have fresh potatoes because for an unknown reason they were never grown on the station; instead, we suffered intensely as we ate our way through tin after tin of the dried variety which looked like coarse breadcrumbs and tasted like chaff.

At that time an entry in my father's diary indicated that one and a half tons of flour had been sent urgently to Barrow Creek in an attempt to save the lives of starving aborigines. But it didn't arrive in time to help all of them:

April 6: Mr Alex McFeat reports from Barrow Creek the

death of three aborigines from starvation.

April 7: Another report from McFeat to say that other aborigines are in a critical condition from starvation.

A fortnight later, on 22nd April 1902, my father recorded that he had sent a telegram to Dr Seabrook at Port Darwin concerning the health of one of our operators, Mr Herbert Koschade. By 26th April his condition had become such that a wire was sent to Dr Marten in Adelaide. That having failed to effect any improvement, and Koschade's health having worsened, my father set out for Oodnadatta on 28th April in the buggy, taking Koschade with him. The last sentence of the entry recording the trip states, "Koschade remained in South Australia."

What the diary doesn't say—and here again I must record the diarist's reticence—is that poor Koschade, a pleasant, amiable young man, laughed endlessly and uncontrollably. At first we thought he may have had a touch of the sun and was mentally upset, but as the days passed and he showed no improvement we knew it to be something far worse than that. I remember seeing him hanging on to a door post and laughing without pause. This went on until we were all nearly frantic with distress. After several days, when he could stand it no longer, my father decided that Koschade would have to be taken to Oodnadatta by buggy. As the officer-in-charge he felt the responsibility for the young man's life was so great that he could not expect anyone else to accept it, so he went alone with him on a nightmare journey of a week to the railhead and then stayed with him in the train for another three days to Adelaide. I remember father telling us when he returned, obviously much the worse for his harrowing experience, that Koschade had laughed from the time he left Alice Springs until they reached Adelaide. A specialist operated to relieve pressure on the brain. Mr Koschade recovered completely, married, raised a family, and died at the age of sixty-eight.

During my brother Mort's illness with diphtheretic paralysis, which I mentioned earlier, my mother had to massage him every morning on the orders of three doctors, telegraphed from the G.P.O. He was then wrapped warmly and made comfortable in the only conveyance we had—a wooden box on wheels—so that he could see what was going on. A special lubra was engaged to look after him, pulling him around in the fresh air all day until gradually he improved. I can see him now, beaming with excitement, supporting himself on his arms on the big dining table as he worked himself around it, swinging his useless legs behind. He recovered completely without any other treatment and, as I've said, died of wounds in France at the age of twenty-four.

Doctor Whitefellow Bradshaw was required to apply his untrained hands to the alleviation of someone's distress almost every week. Fred Raggatt, junior, who stayed with his uncle at one of the Alice Springs stores, was treated for a split forehead and eyebrow after he'd collided with a post while riding. On the third day he'd lost the vision in one eye. My father fixed that with hot fomentations and atropine.

On 4th July 1902, Mr Henry Fitz of Undoolya was riding in the dark when his horse ran into a dead mulga bough which penetrated Mr Fitz's eye. For several days father got pieces of mulga from the wound. Don't I remember that week! Day and night Mr Fitz paced up and down in a darkened room in too much pain to stay still. Again, treatment was prescribed from Adelaide. This included boracic acid, atropine, and finally, when the pain was great, a cocaine lotion. Mr Fitz gradually got better, although he suffered greatly, and eventually made a complete recovery.

And so it went on: Mr T. A. Wallis, senior, was treated with morphia and cinnamon for severe stomach pains which interfered with his breathing, whereas poor Dolly Brookes, the policeman's daughter who had similar symptoms, was given only castor oil.

But I hope I'm not giving the impression that we spent most of our time enduring illnesses and recovering from accidents. Fortunately, the reverse was generally true. Central Australians were a healthy, hardy lot, perhaps because they had to be, and the Bradshaws were among the hardiest of them all. Doctor Whitefellow could hang up his imaginary stethoscope for long enough at least to have time to wonder why it was that his last patient, treated on telegraphed instructions, had recovered so quickly. I sometimes wondered if the thought of being attacked by an amateur frightened the fevers from ailing bodies.

Chapter Eight

VOYAGING VICARS AND OTHER VENERABLES

THERE WERE MANY PLEASANT INTERLUDES during our stay, when interesting travellers made unexpected appearances. All had business to transact at the telegraph station and were glad to combine it with a social visit. For our part, we were always happy to see them; invariably they brought news and gossip that had passed us by. It was from travellers that we learnt new songs and saw the dress and habits of other lands.

On a sunny, but cool, winter afternoon in July 1901, Runge, the senior housegirl, appeared in the doorway of mother's sewing room with an air of excitement, a broad smile on her jolly face...and rather exciting news.

"Quei, more better you bin come see man alonga Boss... him got properly funny feller legs," she said, and screamed with laughter.

They were indeed funny feller legs in that country, for they were clothed in clerical gaiters and belonged to none other than the Right Reverend Gilbert White, Lord Bishop of Carpentaria. In fact his Lordship, with a black frock coat and hat to set off his gaiters, was a novel sight for us as well as for the aborigines. Runge couldn't take her eyes off him. He looked as though he had wandered into our midst by accident or been delivered by the 9.15 whirlwind.

I was only ten years old then, so to me it was a great excitement to have a real Bishop among us. I think he was the first of his kind I'd ever seen and for that to have happened in Alice Springs…well, it seemed to add piquancy to the variety and interest we knew to be ahead of us for a few days.

Bishop White was a middle-aged bachelor, tall, thin, bearded, scholarly, dignified, and, surprisingly, a practical bushman as well as a noted naturalist, like the famous relative after whom he had been named. He was the first bishop of a diocese which had been established only a year earlier, in 1900. This diocese comprised the far northern area of Queensland including the Torres Strait islands, the Gulf of Carpentaria district, and the entire Northern Territory—a total area of three-quarters of a million square miles. It was the largest diocese in Australia and perhaps in the world.

The Bishop's headquarters were (and still are) on Thursday Island, so that when he wanted to visit the few isolated telegraph operators, miners, and pastoralists in Central Australia, who might or might not include some of his parishioners, he had quite a journey ahead of him. First eight hundred miles by sea before he reached Port Darwin, and then a thousand miles overland to Alice Springs. But from the Alice, of course, he had to get back again. His transport between Port Darwin and Alice Springs was arranged by the telegraph stations, each station driving him in a buggy to the next along the line. Subsequently Bishop White had published a record of his remarkable journey which included the following:

"I left Barrow Creek with Mr Bradshaw, the superintendent of the central section of the telegraph line. We had a team of four splendid horses which covered the twenty-two miles to Stirling station in two and a half hours. After dinner we went on to Hanson Well, over sandy country with good grass. The Hanson runs to the north. In this central country the streams seem to run in every direction, but few of them, however large, get anywhere except to run out on sandy flats. Near the well, we saw saltbush for the first time and also a great quantity of parakelia, a succulent plant on which cattle will thrive for a long time without water. In the creek I found an insect-eating plant. It was covered with the bodies of moths and flies...."

As I read Bishop White's story I could see afresh the country in which I had lived for nine years and discover through the eyes of a naturalist much about it that had escaped my notice while I was there.

"We camped at Prowse's Gap, a pass between two ridges of gneissic granite and diorite. [I'd have said, "We camped in the hills."] I climbed up the western ridge and had a most wonderful view...The strata of the ridge here dips almost perpendicularly, forming steep slopes of flat rock. In one of these is a hole about five feet deep and the same length filled with beautiful water; the water follows the dip of the stratum and the hole has apparently been formed by water rushing around pebbles in a crack. These holes are frequent throughout the country but often little known. [See what I mean? The man was a trained observer. He seemed to miss nothing.]

The clearness of the air in these parts is most astonishing. Rocks a quarter of a mile away look almost as if one could lay a hand on them. There is not a particle of haze and the distant mountains stand up with startling clarity.

To my regret we were obliged to travel next day although it was Sunday, there being no water for the horses. [He may have been a scientist but his belief in God was beyond question.] To curtail the journey as much as possible...[apparently to desecrate the Sabbath as little as possible]...we went only six miles after dinner and camped at Native Gap, where I noticed native pines for the first time. We were thus enabled to have a quiet afternoon which I enjoyed after the rush of the last two days. [Rush! Whatever would he say about the pace of today's living? He was averaging less than four miles an hour.]

My Evensong was accompanied by the wild music of the wind in the pines, now swelling into a roar, now dying away into an almost inaudible undertone of sighing. I think that many of the Psalms with the nature voices must have been written in the open air in a land not unlike this in its natural freshness; at any rate they never come so home to one as out in the bush. [What a lovely thought that is. And it could well be so. Listen to the wind in the pines:

He maketh me to lie down in green pastures. He leadeth me beside the still waters.

He restoreth my soul.

The voice of the Lord breaketh the cedars.

The voice of the Lord cleaveth the flames of fire. The voice of the Lord shaketh the wilderness. The voice of the Lord maketh the hinds to calve, And strippeth the forests bare.]

Next day we travelled through dense mulga scrub thirty-five miles to Burt Creek which runs through a little plain 2,300 ft above the sea. [I can almost hear him complaining about the break-neck speed again.]

From the head of the MacDonnell Ranges to Alice Springs are ten miles of as rough a road as I have ever travelled, through low jumbled rocks and ranges, dreary but not unbeautiful. The station itself is surrounded by rocks and must be very hot in summer. At the time of our arrival it was most bitterly cold, and I was devoutly thankful to sleep again in a bed after six days of travelling as cold as any I have ever experienced. Here I found letters, newspapers and other tokens of civilisation although still 322 miles from the railway...I was much interested in the natives here; they have in Mr Bradshaw a courageous and sympathetic sub-protector."

The Bishop's gaiters and heavy black cloth might have been thought to keep him warm, but he complained constantly of the cold. Well, I suppose it was cold.

"Last night the dry bulb went down to between 26 and 27 degrees and the wet bulb to 25 deg. Today I walked up a hill near the station and had a magnificent view. The range, running east and west, has steep walls of rock on the north and south sides, and between them a trough filled with a jumble of low rocky hills. Imagine a great broken sea of yellow water with waves breaking up irregularly with an interval of 200 ft. from the lowest to the highest points, and the foam and broken water all rocks and boulders, and you will have some idea of the scene. All the rocks and stones are yellow and yellowish-red, the grass yellow, and the ground yellow or yellowish-red. Every tint and shade of these colours covers the whole scene, except where it is dotted over the sage green bushes and low stunted trees. The whole blends into a feast of harmonious colours and yet a scene of utter barren desolation. It reminded me strongly...of the deserts and mountains of Palestine. Shape, colour and vegetation seemed to be almost identical, and one was not surprised to see a camel team threading its way through one of the narrow defiles by which the rivers find their way to the south.

I have never seen anything quite like these gaps. Heavitree Gap, through which the south road [sic] passes, is a gap in the range about one hundred yards wide entirely filled by the sandy bed of the River Todd, along which the road also passes. [Today the highway, the railway, the river, and the telegraph line all pass through the Gap.] The cliffs on either side are a slatey reddishyellow sandstone with the strata very distinct and tilted at an angle of 45 degrees. They rise abruptly to a height of 200 ft. Just to the south of the gap is a lately discovered hot spring on the top of a low mound. No water is visible but a gentle steam rises covering the stones with moss and condensing on the under sides of the stones in drops of dew. The rock is limestone mixed with igneous ironstone and surrounded by granite."

There wasn't much he didn't know!

The Bishop spent most of his week with us exploring and making sketches of the hills around the station. In the evenings he and my father settled down to a solemn game of chess. For such a ceremony as chess, said to be the most scientific of all games, there had to be complete silence. We children were banished and not allowed within earshot. Mother and the governess were glared at if they so much as whispered. They bore it nobly as long as they could; but one night they caught each other's eye, then choked and fled, followed by baleful looks from father and a mildly surprised inquiring look from the Bishop as much as to say, "Good gracious! Whatever can be the matter with the ladies?"

His Lordship was very interested in a large box of rubies— more correctly, garnets—left behind by the Gillens. They had been found in the ranges years before in large quantities and were of no great value. The Bishop thought he'd like to have some made up as a gift for his sister, so the children got busy and washed a few handfuls of the stones, which were then spread on a mirror in the sunlight, thus making it easy to choose those with the best colour.

Years later we met Gilbert White again at Port Pirie when he was the first Bishop of Willochra. He told us then that the stones, polished and set, had made a beautiful ornament.

On the Sunday he was with us (4th August 1901) we all attended a morning service he conducted at the station. "It was a great joy after all the weeks in the bush to hear the canticles sung again, and sung well," he wrote. Sing-songs, as I've said, were one of our chief diversions, so I would have been surprised if he hadn't complimented us.

> "Mister Bradshaw, since his coming, has held service every Sunday for his family and those of the telegraph station and township who like to attend. *O si sic omnes!* After Matins a celebration of Holy Communion, with five communicants. It was delightful to celebrate the Divine Mysteries here for the first time in the centre of Australia and to feel at one with the congregation of the Cathedral of the Diocese 1,800 miles away. In the afternoon we had a service at the township, and our congregation consisted of all the adult population except two. We had a most hearty service, singing all the canticles and some beautiful hymns. It was many a long year since most of the congregation had last attended service and it seemed to be thoroughly appreciated by all.
>
> I left Alice Springs and my kind hosts with great regret. Everyone was more than kind and the country is, I think, the most interesting and in some ways the most beautiful I have seen in Australia. I was the only passenger on the mail coach to Oodnadatta... We passed a train of twenty-five camels with loading for Alice Springs. They are curious snakey-looking beasts as they slide along in single file...Driving through this country is really a sinecure as the driver simply straps the reins to the seat and reads the paper, or indulges in such sleep as

a driver may without being too far gone to objurgate the horses from time to time. Ours were always being promised a tremendous thrashing a few yards further on, but it never came for they were excellent horses and most excellently driven. The driver at last convulsed me by exclaiming pathetically as we toiled slowly through a slough of sand, `Get on, you nasty things; what would King Edward say if he could see his coach going at such a rate?' "

Well, that convulsed us, too. The driver, Tom Williams, was renowned from Oodnadatta to Barrow Creek for his colourful language. On mail days, while the coach was still toiling through Middle Park and the river below us, we could hear, from a mile away, Tom's personal opinion of the team and what he'd like to do to them. His vituperation was generally the signal for the cry of "Mail-oh! I can hear Tom Williams swearing." But he must have been overawed by the Bishop's clerical dress, or by his very presence, to have descended to such mild epithets as "nasty things."

The sandhills seemed to take some of the steam out of Gilbert White the naturalist, which didn't surprise me. They appalled him:

"The sandhills are endless. We toil up one only to find an exactly similar one ahead. Only very staunch horses could possibly pull the coach through. Next day we toiled for miles through the famous Depot Sandhills. The mail is allowed two days for the twenty-six miles between Alice Well and Horseshoe Bend, and no wonder! I should think four miles a day, two in the morning and two in the afternoon, about a fair thing. But our powerful horses did about two miles an hour with great exertion. Some of the hills are high and steep even for firm ground, and all are covered with sand three to six feet deep. We camped in the bed of the Finke River. A cold night and no shelter. In the morning, ice two inches thick was on the dishes.

A few miles further on we came to Horseshoe Bend and there met the northbound coach."

The Bishop, alas, left the Centre with a bad last impression:

"There were a dozen men all more or less drunk, chiefly more. I had a tiny room about six feet square which I offered to share with one of the north-bound passengers who had accidentally shot himself in the leg and was afraid of being injured by some of the drunken men. There were two fights during the night and plenty of quarrelling, while the language was enough to set the place on fire. I was glad to walk on my way next morning and let the coach overtake me…"

His Lordship was not amused, and I can't say I blamed him.

It was some years later—in 1907—that another pair of funny feller legs appeared on the station.

They weren't funny; they were downright hilarious, and we had to be extremely careful where and when we laughed, and at whom.

There had been a succession of visitors—prospectors, government surveyors, officers from the Indian Army looking for cheap remounts, a few drifters, a few labourers, and a few builders (the population was still only about twelve Europeans when we left a year later but they were building a substantial gaol, just in case) . More often than not the coach from Oodnadatta arrived without passengers at all. But then one day there came from the north the kind of diversion which made our long, unchanging days worth while and, comparatively speaking, turned the station into what might have been an annexe of Bedlam.

Runge came in and announced the newcomer's arrival with the statement, "Him got funny feller trouser different-way." We interpreted that as meaning he was like the Bishop, only different.

And different he was. The funny feller trouser belonged

to a funny feller man—a Rumanian globe-trotter who, accompanied by only one aboriginal and a packhorse, had ridden a thousand miles from Port Darwin through an utterly strange land, making it obvious that his addiction to travel must have been strong indeed. He was wearing a Norfolk deer-stalker suit of the largest and loudest checks I had ever seen. The funny feller trousers were really plusfours tucked into long socks at the knee, the first of their kind, I'm sure, ever to have seen Central Australian sunlight. They were certainly the first the natives had seen; they gaped in astonishment and giggled behind their hands, but then raced for the sanctuary of the camp to add to the raucous bellowing already emanating from those there who had seen the new arrival.

He was Monsieur Constantin Statesco, a member of a unique European explorers' club of which both the Emperor of Austria and the German Kaiser were patrons. I suppose it was a forerunner of the geographical societies of today. Every year three members of the club set out on a world tour; in 1907, in Australia at least, that might well have been regarded as exploring, especially if the way M. Statesco tackled matters was any criterion for the others. Each of them wrote a paper on what he saw but never touched on politics. Where it was possible they had to travel on foot, but in some countries— where distances were great and time an important factor they were allowed to supplement their two feet with the four of a horse. Australia was one such country. M. Statesco reported to us that of the two men who set out with him one had died and the other had found compelling reasons to return home; so of that year's crop he was the only survivor. He carried a document to be attested to by a magistrate at each place he visited; as my father was away I don't know who filled that role in Alice Springs.

The stoutness of M. Statesco's heart and the durability of his flesh was unfortunately not matched by the adequacy of his English. All he knew had been picked up on the sea trip between the Philippines and Port Darwin; after that his black boy had continued the good teaching work—and how! I still blush when I think of it.

The poor man was most distressed when one of the men broke the news to him that his language would not be tolerated in the salons of Paris or Bucharest and it wasn't going to be tolerated in Alice Springs. Fifty per cent of his English consisted of awful swear words he had learnt from the natives, and he used them with a continental flourish of the hands that gave them terrible emphasis.

"You tell de ladies...please tell dem...I did not know...I did not understand," he protested, and we knew that he really didn't.

Poor M. Statesco. He came at the most disorganized time I recall. My father was visiting Adelaide. There had been a serious breakdown on the O.T. Line and some of the men were away attending to it. That meant the operators remaining on the station had to be glued to their instruments day and night. To make matters worse, we were without a governess for the first time since our arrival eight years earlier. Miss Mabel Taylor had gone and there just weren't any takers for the position; either the Australian spirit of adventure was waning or governesses had discovered the value of money and wanted more than my father was able to pay. That meant I was left with the responsibility of teaching the younger members of the family with the knowledge that had been passed on to me by four governesses. I was then only sixteen, but I taught English, arithmetic, history, geography, and a little French to Mort, Consie, and Jack. Scarcely anyone on the station except the natives—and he was now scared of them—had time to talk to or entertain our visitor. He endured a lonely fortnight that must

The main street of Alice Springs (Stuart it was then)

Barrow Creek telegraph station, where two men were speared to death in 1874

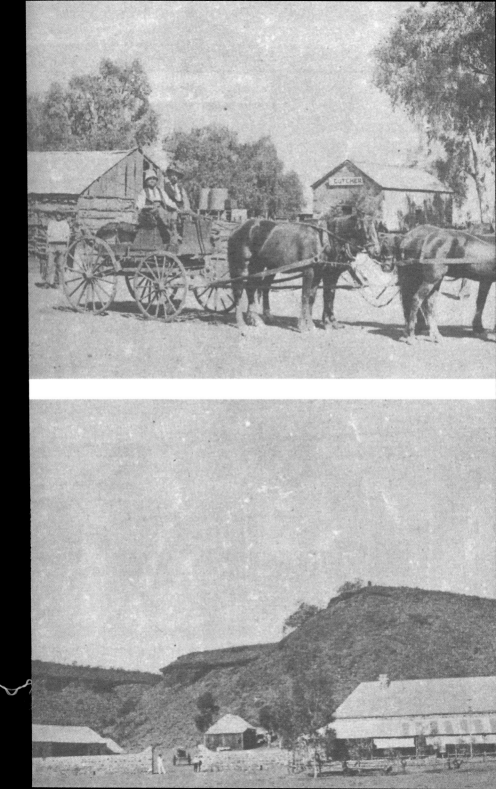

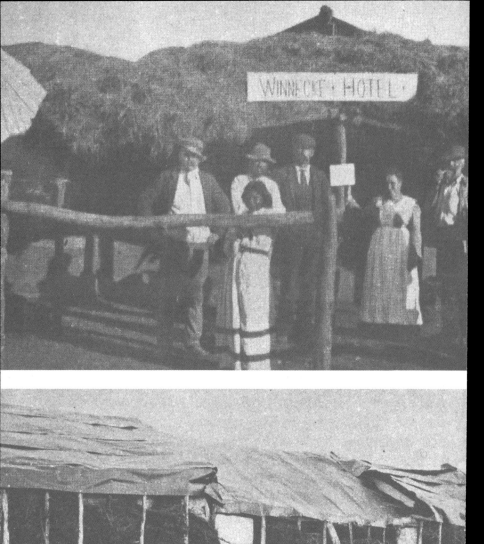

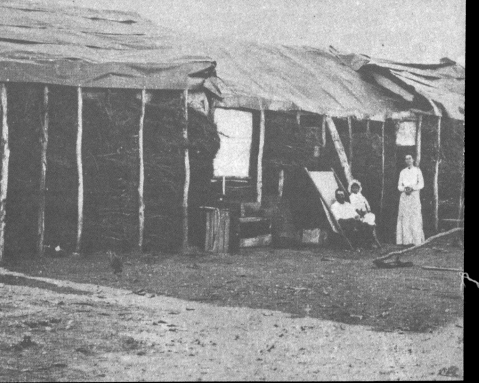

have seemed like a year in a foreign land where his knowledge of the language consisted mainly of offensive words.

One day he was persuaded to play tennis with Arthur Kunoth, Harry's brother, on the very first court to be built in Alice Springs. But that was a washout; the bindy-eyes lay around the court in thousands. Each time the Rumanian picked up a ball that had gone into the grass he complained bitterly about his handful of "preekles." Matters weren't improved because Arthur had recruited a cheer-squad of aboriginal boys for himself, leaving his opponent friendless. Each time Arthur hit the ball the boys shouted "Hooray for Arthur," as instructed; but when M. Statesco hit a winner it was received in silence. That must have had a depressing effect on him and his visage grew daily gloomier.

Mother was sorry for him and one night asked if he would care to join us for tea. Father was still away, but she thought he might like to share a meal with our family after more than a week with the men at the mercy of the cook's boiled beef. For a man who had been accustomed to gilded halls and continental cuisine this must have represented diabolical torture, but I gathered that the trip was self-inflicted, so he had nobody to blame but himself. He accepted our invitation with an eagerness that made his suffering obvious and prepared suitably for the auspicious occasion—or so he thought. But imagine the futile attempts to hide our giggles when he appeared in a formal dinner suit. In Alice Springs!

"I have changed," he announced, noticing that nobody else had.

That was one of the understatements of the year. He was utterly resplendent in stiff white shirt, black dinner suit, a bow tie, and patent leather shoes. How he managed to carry it all

Winnecke Hotel, a log, rail, and tent inn of 1904

Living-it-up, Central Australian style, 1906. Mr and Mrs George Lines outside their home at Winnecke goldfield

on horseback was a mystery we never solved, but I suppose every European gentleman worthy of the name must be prepared to change into a dinner jacket on those occasions when is invited out—even though he's been invited only from the men's quarters to the house next door in the middle of an unexplored continent.

Mother's brother, Ernest Allchurch, had come to Alice Springs some time before to join the staff of operators. He had married at Hermannsburg and lived with his wife in a small log cottage on the station. Mother felt that somehow or other she had to acknowledge the tribute M. Statesco had paid us by "changing." So I was sent to plead with Uncle Ernest and Aunt Bessie to come over, and to beg Aunt Bessie, if necessary, to bring her songs.

Well, we did our best, but shocking inferiority complexes and the language barrier rather cramped our style. The going was heavy. I admired the delicate green of the sky after a beautiful sunset. Constantin sighed and gazed nostalgically at it, murmuring something about "Payee, ah Paree at this hour! De lights, de carriages, de theatre, de lovely ladies," which might have been taken as an insult by the ladies present—but wasn't. Then he told us about the latest hit tune from the boulevards…it was rocking Paris when he was last there, he said, and of course we wouldn't know it but it went something like this....

"Oh, you mean 'After the Ball is Over', " Aunt Bessie said, and sang it for him.

"Surely not the latest hit in Paris?" she asked, a little archly. "Why, Queen Victoria and Prince Albert sang that—it was one of their favourites."

As might be expected, Constantin produced his family photographs and showed them around, explaining that his father was a "clergyman" of justice. Later we discovered he was the Rumanian Minister of Justice.

He had some beautiful gifts from famous people: a gold cigarette holder from the Mikado, a ruby from the Emperor of Abyssinia, and silver from the King of Siam. His present from the Russians was a gaol sentence in Siberia, until released on the intervention of various foreign consuls. The Russo-Japanese war had ended only a year before, following the destruction of the Russian Fleet at the Battle of Tsushima. Japanese nationals were not the most loved persons in Russia, and M. Statesco, through no fault of his own, certainly looked like one. He had black hair, and olive skin, and he was slightly almond-eyed from some earlier infusion of Oriental blood.

The Alice Springs climate or the moonlight must have affected him, too, for one day he copied from a magazine a sentimental poem entitled "Spring" and presented it to me. It was apt, he said, because "Spring...you know...Alice Spring." He told mother it was high time I was married—at sixteen— and went so far as to select for me a suitable husband from the limited raw material on the station.

Unfortunately his selection turned out to be one who already had a wife and family in Adelaide.

At a time when M. Statesco was beginning to wear a little thin we were thankful for the arrival of the mail coach with Tom Williams in the driver's seat. Having disposed of his horses, the Rumanian was "taking passage," as they say, with Tom, who would have the pleasure of his company for a week or more. Constantin arrived at the appointed departure time immaculately dressed for the road in his deer-stalker plus-fours. Tom looked at the loud checks doubtfully and opened his mouth to speak—I'm sure it would have been a strong epithet—but then realized there were ladies present. I'll bet that he had improved Constantin's vocabulary by the time they reached Oodnadatta. Apart from being the most fluid and vitriolic swearer anywhere north of Adelaide, Tom was a surprisingly good Shakespearian scholar; he would thus have put a classical polish on the foundation of cursing laid by the blackboy.

Chapter Nine

THE SMOKING BUGGY

THE MAIN NORTH ROAD, THE ONLY ONE, THEN passed through the telegraph station a few yards from my room. I therefore think it deserves capital letters, even though it has since changed both its route and its name and become the Stuart Highway.

Along it, one day in December 1907, came travellers who caused more excitement among the whites and more panic among the blacks than anything else during our stay there.

Natives rushed to the station office with the news that on the track a few hundred yards away there was a "buggy going all by hisself, him got smoke coming out Tonga him." We showed little consternation, and that perplexed them, but it was only because we had advance word from telegraph stations to the south that Mr Harry Dutton, of Anlaby, Kapunda, and his colleague, Mr Murray Aunger, were on the way in the first motor car to attempt to cross Australia.

We had seen one or two of these horseless carriages in Adelaide during a holiday in 1904, so we knew what to expect in a physical sense as well. I had even had a ride in one at Glene1g. In those days riding in a car was roughly the same as riding in an aeroplane in the 1930s and in a space capsule in the 1960s. I remember that it had high seats arranged back to back, which meant a hair-raising experience for the rear seat passengers. But to most of the men in Alice Springs at that time the car was a novelty, the first they had seen, and the natives couldn't have been more terrified of the Devil himself.

The camp on the river bank broke into pandemonium. I've never seen such panic: elderly lubras, clasping their precious dogs, scrambled up trees like teenagers, making sure that they would be well out of range of the smoking monster if it should come their way: infectious dread spread among hundreds of mangy dogs which howled piteously; piccaninnies cowered or yelled with fright. But finally almost every soul on the station came to stare and wonder and give a welcome to the first motorists, while keeping their escape routes open in case the monstrous thing should belch and roar as it had on arrival.

Thirty or so horses in the stockyard were as frightened as the natives and galloped around madly; one, shut in the small breaking-in yard, jumped the six feet high rail fence, raced westwards, and wasn't found until many days later.

Only the old men of the tribe, the Aranda Elders, were unmoved, or pretended to be. I suppose they had to put on a brave face in front of the others. They glanced disdainfully at the smoking buggy and then returned to their accustomed contemplation of the surrounding tribal land.

Les Spicer, one of the operators, asked an old patriarch named Billy what he thought of the car.

Billy thought about the question for a long time. Then he spat disgustedly, albeit eloquently, and said, "I reckon might-be that white-feller properly Number-One fool. Him make'im anything like buggy-longa-smoke. But he can't make'im rain, eh?" And that was that.

The car was a 24-horse-power Talbot that had been built in England. It was devoid of mudguards, but had a high box body festooned with spare tyres, shovels, axes, rifles, water bags, a windlass, coils of matting, brass acetylene headlamps, and a bulbous horn. On 25th November 1907, when it was farewelled from the Adelaide G.P.O. by a curious crowd, no car had been farther north than Hawker. The country beyond that was known only by the cattle drovers, the mail-coachmen, the camel teamsters, and the few souls like ourselves who had gone into the wilderness because that was where we were sent or taken.

Fourteen years after that epic trip began, Geoffrey Dutton, the well-known author and lecturer, was born at Kapunda.

Fifty-one years after his father and Murray Aunger first made the trip, Geoffrey Dutton, his elder brother John, and James Gosse, drove a Talbot to Darwin again. It wasn't the original car, which didn't get right through, but a second one that had been imported specially from England and had completed the journey in 1908.

Geoffrey Dutton tells us that months of careful preparation were necessary before the first trip could begin. How many people today realize the difficulties? There were no garages or bowsers, so petrol had to be sent out by train and camel and dumped at appropriate distances along the track. The car itself was fitted with special equipment such as Stepney wheels which could be bolted to the outside of the existing wheel to give greater traction in soft sand. The Michelin tyres were steel-studded. The car and equipment weighed two and a half tons.

This all happened at a time when interstate travel by car was chiefly along bush tracks. A Talbot had just broken the Melbourne—Sydney record at an average speed of 28 m.p.h., and the Adelaide—Melbourne record stood at something over 28 hours.

Dutton and Aunger were not attempting to break a record; they were really on a journey of exploration for the introduction of the motor-driven wheel to places it had never previously penetrated.

"Impossible," the sceptics said.

"We'll do it," Harry Dutton said, and he did. But, frankly, I'd rather have walked or gone in a buggy.

Cars were still so scarce in 1907 that when Dutton and Aunger left the Adelaide G.P.O. they created a sensation. Several hundred people gathered to wave them goodbye. A contemporary newspaper account said that "Mr Dutton took the seat at the steering pillar...and the car was set in motion..."

Within six days they were at Coward Springs, north of Marree, where they encountered the first disaster. The bulk of the petrol so carefully sent forward had been left in the sun for several months and the intense heat had burst the flimsy tins. They had to go by train to Oodnadatta, the terminus of the railway, where the next fuel dump had been established.

Harry Dutton had christened the car "Angelina," but it wouldn't be surprising if she were called a few other names on what must have been a truly fearful trip. A week after leaving Oodnadatta they ran into the worst obstacle so far, the wide sandy bed of the Alberga River, with steep banks on either side. Great ingenuity and perseverance were needed to get across. The plan was to inspect several likely crossings before selecting the best, unloading the car, and carrying all equipment through the sand to the far bank in order to lighten the load. That took three hours! Then slowly Angelina heaved her way across the quarter-mile of dry sand, with the temperature at 113 in the shade. That day Dutton and Aunger covered 40 miles. We could do as well with our horse-drawn buggy, and often did.

They reached Blood's Creek the next day and there the country changed to rough gibber plain—hard, but excellent going for the car. Yet they had been warned by the station manager that this would be a tough stretch. At first the two men were baffled by these reports of the country ahead.

"What's the road like?"

"Why, wonderful…easy going," the drovers would say.

But the motorists would find themselves struggling through soft sand. "Terrible going," on the other hand, invariably turned out to be gibber country where they made excellent time. Of course, the drovers were thinking in terms of hoofs rather than wheels.

When Dutton and Aunger crossed the South Australian border at Charlotte Waters the mere fact of being in the Northern Territory made Darwin seem closer. But I knew what was ahead of them once they entered the beautiful sandhills… beautiful, that is, to anyone but a motorist. In a bad creek nine miles from Charlotte Waters they bogged so deeply that they had to stay there overnight and work Angelina through it on a Spanish windlass.

The next obstacle was the Finke River with its broad bed of sand that had to be crossed five times. But there was worse than that to come—the dreaded Depot Sandhills were between Horseshoe Bend and Alice Well. Some were sixty feet high with grades of one in three. Our horses had grunted and struggled to take us through in winter. I can only imagine the torture that these two men, and Angelina as well, must have suffered trying to get through in summer with the sand too hot to touch.

Although the auxiliary Stepney wheels were bolted on, the sand failed to provide traction and the wheels spun at a terrific speed, creating miniature whirlwinds. They couldn't hope to get through and finally enlisted the aid of a team of donkeys. Harry Dutton must have been staggered by the sight of donkeys pulling what was then one of the finest cars in the world. Even with the donkeys, however, steering was extremely difficult and sand backed right up to the seat. There were thirteen sandhills in four miles, and of the twenty-five miles from Horseshoe Bend to Alice Well there was hard surface for only two hundred yards. Only thirteen of the last seventy miles into Alice Springs were on firm ground. In spite of these conditions, Angelina gave no trouble at all. Incredibly, she had drunk only one pint of water since leaving Adelaide.

We were all very pleased to have Mr Dutton and Mr Aunger with us, but they remained for only one day before resuming their contact with the privations of the "road" that beggared description. However, those who have been to Kapunda and seen what the Duttons have done at Anlaby will realize that no member of the family would be easily deterred by a rough track.

On 16th December 1907 they set out through the MacDonnell Ranges along a boulder-strewn path that no modern motorist would tackle except in a four-wheel drive vehicle. Once through the hills they struck the best going since leaving Quorn and by nightfall had covered 133 miles, having remained constantly alert for mulga stumps and anthills hidden in the long grass. At this stage, when they had travelled more than half the distance and would now apparently rush through to Darwin, the weather turned against them. Rain began to fall in earnest. They were held up at Barrow Creek for four days and did not leave for Tennant Creek until three days before Christmas. Already it was too late. The dry soil had turned to red mud, the creeks into lakes and swamps. Faithful Angelina's transmission began to feel the strain of endless revving and grinding through bogs. Finally the yoke of the universal joint split and it was obvious that a temporary repair would be useless. That, it seemed, was that.

There was nothing for it but to abandon the trip. They threw a wire over the telegraph line, as the station operators had asked them to do if they struck serious trouble, and waited for a rescue party. It wasn't long in coming, paradoxically hauled by three or four horse-power where the twenty-four horse-power of the motor car had failed. Meanwhile they had plenty of food and were surrounded by water, and there was time to contemplate the long drive back to Oodnadatta in a buggy.

If anyone thought that initial failure was likely to deter Harry Dutton and Murray Aunger they didn't know either gentleman. Back at Anlaby, Dutton cabled at once to England for the latest 25 h.p. model Talbot, slightly more powerful than Angelina and with a floating rear axle more suited to the punishment ahead of it. I was one of those who was wrong. I remember the travellers arriving back at Alice Springs in the station buggy. They were bearded and dirty and downcast and, I thought, defeated. But like John McDouall Stuart, who had to make three attempts before crossing the continent in 1862, their enthusiasm for the task in hand had only been whetted. Mr Dutton's determination can be gauged from the fact that he was paying the expenses himself; unlike McDouall Stuart, he wasn't subsidized by the government. And it must have cost him thousands of pounds.

By 30th June, 1908, they were on their way again, complete with spare parts for Angelina, who had spent a lonely few months north of Barrow Creek. At least they had learnt respect for the weather and now travelled in mid-winter. With the more powerful engine they got over the Depot Sandhills with less difficulty and by the end of July were approaching Tennant Creek. We had the pleasure of seeing them at Alice Springs for the second time on 22nd July, less than one month before the Bradshaw family's long exile in Central Australia ended. On 11th August we set out in the station buggy for Oodnadatta and reached there fourteen days later, having averaged five miles an hour. In nine years our speed hadn't increased by as much as one mile an hour; and this time we had motor tracks on our trail to remind us that there now really was a faster means of travel than a horse-drawn buggy.

But you think we had a tough trip? Why, in the very year we left, Fred Blakely and brothers Jim and Dick O'Neil rode push-bikes from South Australia to Darwin. A dog named Jethro accompanied them all the way, sometimes trotting beside his masters, sometimes sitting on the handlebars or in a box over the rear wheels. Blakely and the O'Neill carried their own bedrolls around their shoulders and chests like military bandoliers; apart from that they had nothing and apparently wanted nothing. They were prospectors who were at home anywhere in the bush. Distance didn't worry them; they pedalled on and on, day after day, week after week, stopping beside the track when they were tired or felt like stopping or wanted to boil the billy. They called at the telegraph station, having carried their bikes through the Depot Sandhills, just as Dutton and Aunger were preparing to leave. I remember that the horseless carriage had seemed to us a difficult way of travelling through the trackless desert, but whatever hardships the drivers had were overshadowed by the experiences of Blakeley and his friends. Nor were they the only ones to ride bikes through the Centre to Darwin. It had also been done by Francis Birtles, Ted Reichenbach, and J. Murif.

When Dutton and Aunger left Alice Springs on their second trip they took today's equivalent of a wireless transmitter with them in case of trouble. This was my uncle, Ernest Allchurch, who carried equipment to tap the telegraph line. They found Angelina exactly as she'd been left, untouched after seven months in the centre of Australia. She must undoubtedly have been not only the loneliest car in the world, but the one least likely to be stolen. If Dutton and Aunger couldn't shift her it was certain that nobody could. She had been the subject of aboriginal speculation, but they apparently were terrified of approaching too closely.

In any case, they had been utterly baffled by the dotted track the steel-studded tyres had made.

Angelina's tyres were still partially inflated and the engine started immediately. The universal joint was replaced and the men left in the strangest convoy ever to go that way, Dutton driving his old love, Angelina, and Aunger the new car. The going was relatively easy for two hundred miles to Newcastle Waters, except for the constant menace of rockhard anthills hidden in the long grass. They knew that if one of these punctured a sump they would again be in serious trouble, but that didn't happen.

Their next big problem was to cross the Sturt Plain, seventeen miles of cracked black soil north of Newcastle Waters. It was covered in high grass with ruts up to two feet deep for the whole distance. As might be imagined, this was ferociously severe on springs and wheels, sometimes making it almost impossible to steer. At one point, they covered only five miles in three hours. Then came thick scrub, which the leading car plunged through like a scrub-roller, flattening small trees and bushes before it. Dry coolibah swamps repeated the jolting near Dunmara. Occasionally the two drivers were thrown bodily from their seats. Poor old Angelina's body had to be roped to the chassis.

Then there was another hazard. Near Daly Waters the aborigines were burning the long grass to help them in their hunting. By doing so they frightened game which ran towards them...and their spears. For many miles the country was alight and it seemed that there was a good chance of incineration. But the motorists took the chance and raced into Daly Waters, their lungs filled with smoke and the cars covered with burning ash and leaves. On these sections, of course, there were no hotels or motels, certainly no breakfast pushed to them through a slot. They rolled out their swags and camped beside the vehicles, brewing tea and eating salt beef.

In the Centre they'd had difficulty with sandhills, but north of Daly Waters and Katherine water became the chief problem. Dozens of creeks and rivers had to be forded and a few of them were bridged. The ford over the Edith River, for instance, was four feet deep with a strong current. Dutton and Aunger tied tarpaulins over the front of the cars and drove them flat out into the water, making a bow wave that swept twenty to thirty feet up the far bank. Angelina stopped six feet from the bank, but the second car got clean across. There were other problems, but no doubt existed then that they would get to Darwin. They did—on 20th August 1908, after 2,100 miles and 42 travelling days—and thus became the first motorists to cross the continent. There was great delight in Adelaide and the event was hailed there as the most important so far in "automobilism" in Australia. The front axles of both cars were bent and the bodies showed wear and tear, but neither had given mechanical trouble. Even more amazing is the fact that they had only three punctures from hidden stakes though they drove constantly through open bush.

Old Angelina has long since disappeared, but the second Talbot is still in the Anlaby garage. For many years she ran into Kapunda from Anlaby to pick up mail and stores; then, until the jubilee trip, she went into honourable retirement. But it wouldn't be surprising if Geoffrey Dutton's sons take her from the stables at Anlaby in the year 2008 and follow the trail of their father and grandfather to Darwin. I hope so. And I also hope that they let the old girl see again the site of her brief stay at the Alice Springs telegraph station, which is now a museum.

One museum piece visiting another, so to speak.

Our visitors had arrived with increasing frequency, but this was the only horseless carriage we saw until our return to Adelaide.

One of the travellers we saw several times was Dr Charles Chewings, an Adelaide geologist and anthropologist, whose name has been perpetuated in Alice Springs. He was a colourful personality and we always enjoyed seeing him, though my mother might have been happier had he been a doctor of medicine instead of a doctor of philosophy. During one of his visits a man from an outback station went on a drinking spree at the Stuart Arms Hotel, leaving his unfortunate horse tied up outside. (This is one facet of cruelty to animals that has disappeared since cars replaced horses.) When he finally staggered out and tried to mount, the horse expressed its disgust with a vicious kick that almost knocked the man's ear off.

As usual, father was sent for. Being the senior government official, it was apparently presumed that he knew more about such matters than others; either that, or his reputation had been inflated since he fixed Harry Dixon's broken thigh.

My father enlisted a number of burly men to act as nurses. Their only task was to sit on the man and hold him still while the amateur surgeon went to work with needle and thread from my mother's sewing basket.

I suppose the poor patient couldn't be blamed for his language. Throughout the painful proceedings he abused my father unmercifully, and likened his delicate embroidery to that of a sewer of wheat bags.

"Where's Chewings?" he demanded constantly. "Go and get him! What the deuce is the good of having a doctor in the place if I can't have him sew me up."

I'm sure Doctor Chewings knew less about such matters than my father but his patient wouldn't be convinced. He deserved to get tetanus but was so tough that I doubt whether he even had a good headache; if he did, it was more likely to have been caused by his hangover than the kick from the horse.

My father dressed the wound with cotton wool, bandaged it, and told him not to touch it for a while. The man grumbled again, mounted his horse, returned the kick it had given him, and then rode back to his station, most ungrateful and firmly convinced that he'd been shabbily treated.

A fortnight later someone saw him in the bush with the cotton-wool bandage still untouched. It was filthy and should obviously have set up an infection. Horrified, the traveller removed the bandage, cleaned the wound, and later reported that the ear was as good as new.

"A trifle crooked perhaps, but it's difficult to notice," he said.

Other mining experts came and went on their way to the goldfields at Arltunga or farther north, men whose names were well known at the time but have since been forgotten. And there was the usual crop of odd characters who seem to be inseparable from the outback, perhaps absconders from justice or debt or nagging wives. They'd drift into Alice Springs on the mail coach, or sometimes on foot, and disappear again as quickly as they'd come, following their own mysterious business.

There was a home missionary named Albert Lennox who seemed to spend his entire life on walkabout through the Northern Territory but never carried enough water with him. He was forever being rescued from the brink of death but would then go off at once and repeat the performance. He was a constant worry to my father and the other operators who kept a kindly telegraphic eye on all such travellers, reporting them "in" and "out" from the various stations along the line, passing the responsibility for their care from one to the other until they finally reached civilization.

From dates in the diary it appears that Mr Lennox rode from Port Darwin to Oodnadatta in 1900. His funds must have been at rock-bottom and he lived as best he could accepting meals and shelter from the kind-hearted people along the track. There must have been times when he didn't eat for several days or perhaps a week, but like a camel with water he seemed able to eat and store food against the time when his body needed it; presumably it was then released into the bloodstream, thus providing the energy for him to go on.

There was one occasion, following three days at the telegraph station, when Mr Lennox took his leave after breakfast. That should be more accurately written as "after breakfasts." He had a meal of meat, vegetables, and coffee with the operators in their dining room at 7.30. He bid them a quick goodbye and was in time to join us for our breakfast, which was also a hearty one. But that wasn't all; our subsequent gossip revealed that while passing through the township he called to say goodbye to Mrs Charlie Meyers. Now I'm not suggesting that a man of God would tell Mrs Meyers a lie, but surely she would have asked him whether or not he'd had breakfast, and in any case she'd expect that we would have fed him before such a long trip. Nevertheless, Mr Lennox somehow managed to convey that he hadn't broken his fast and was given another meal there. Mrs Meyers could have been pardoned for thinking that the hospitality at the telegraph station was slipping. Fancy letting a poor man start out for Oodnadatta without a substantial meal! And what must Mrs Charles Brookes have thought at the Heavitree Gap police station when he arrived there soon afterwards and accepted breakfast from her? Our inquiries showed that the owner of this gargantuan appetite had eaten four big meals in less than two hours. In any case, it was enough to carry him to Charlotte Waters which he reached six days later.

A sigh of relief is almost evident in the last entry in my father's diary which deals with that visit of Mr Lennox. It said simply: "Lennox reached Oodnadatta." That meant he would go aboard the train for Adelaide, and thus pass from the responsibility of the O.T. Line and its officers.

But don't imagine that that was the last we saw of him. Oh, no; he came back all right, and, as had been predicted, he died of thirst one torrid summer in the wilds north of Alice Springs.

Another lone ranger who appeared on the station had declined the offer of a ride by the mailman over the last stage from Alice Well to Alice Springs.

"I'm in a hurry," he explained.

Whether or not the mailman took that as an insult isn't recorded, but the fact is that the traveller beat the mail to the station by three hours. On his arrival, my uncle Ernest Allchurch asked if he'd walked all the way from Adelaide.

"Oh, no!" he said, a trifle indignantly. "I took the train to Gawler."

Gawler is 25 miles north of Adelaide, so at least he had saved himself one-fortieth part of the thousand miles walk to Alice Springs. After resting for a few days he walked through to Port Darwin, worked there for three months, then walked all the way back to Adelaide.

"I didn't like the place," he explained. The operators along the line who were checking him in and out for the best part of a year could be pardoned for thinking that he was slightly deranged.

Among our most welcome visitors were the Line Party. Day-to-day maintenance of the O.T. Line had to be done by the local linemen and as I've said often by the operators themselves. In addition, it was patrolled regularly by a party of experts who arrived in a laden wagon hauled by ten horses. They were responsible for the permanent maintenance of poles, insulators, and wires on the 800-mile section between Oodnadatta and Powell Creek. We saw them twice a year on their way north and again on the return trip to Oodnadatta.

They were a lively crew, all expert Bushmen and horsemen; they had to be to survive in that country. During our stay the man most frequently in charge was Tom Hanley, a tall, self-reliant bushie who, I'm sure, could have driven around Australia in his wagon. He had gone to Peake telegraph station west of Lake Eyre as a lad. Peake survives on today's maps only as a river bed which in the occasional wet season runs and spills its contents into the Neales and eventually Lake Eyre. But when Tom Hanley first went there it was the most northerly telegraph station. Like Strangways and Blood's Creek and Charlotte Waters, it was an important stopping place on the overland track before the railway went through to Oodnadatta, passing it by and allowing it to be forgotten. However the journals of the early explorers like Ernest Giles and the early missionaries like Kempe and Schwarz attest to its original importance as a staging camp. For Kempe and Schwarz, who established the Finke River mission at Hermannsburg in 1877 after a journey that lasted two years, Peake was an oasis they reached in dire circumstances. They had two thousand sheep and other stock, and still had to face the desert crossing in temperatures that ranged up to 126 degrees. Little wonder they regarded it as a haven, the last point from which they could communicate by telegram with their people in Adelaide.

Hanley was one of the O.T. Line's most experienced bushmen. He had ridden along the route in 1870 with the survey parties, and he went with Ernest Giles on his westerly penetration from Lake Eyre through the Great Victorian Desert. I've wished many times that I had then been old enough to leave on record the stories that Tom Hanley and other Inlanders like Alex Ross told us on their visits to the station. Alas, I didn't do it; I didn't think of doing it because what they told us really wasn't so extraordinary at the time. How was I to know that within a few years the stories of their adventures and privations would be forgotten with the advent of the motorized wheel, the formed road, the radio, and the other technological advances that have taken the danger—and perhaps the spice—from life in the outback.

The story of Tom Hanley's life might have been a classic of Australian literature, but he took it with him to his grave.

Chapter Ten

THE CANTANKEROUS COUNTRY

WHAT A CANTANKEROUS AND UNPREDICTABLE country it is! One day we were in the grip of what appeared to be an everlasting drought. Within 24 hours we were needing an ark rather than a buggy to get us through the flooded land.

One day the only mineral in sight was the micaceous glitter in the earth. Next week we had a gold rush on our hands!

For some years gold had been mined at Arltunga. Several hundred pounds worth was shipped south unescorted on the fortnightly mail coach. Precautions against theft were not taken because none were needed; anyone who robbed the coach could not hope to escape in a land where the wells were thirty miles apart and led inevitably to the policeman in the nearest town.

Then, in 1902, a rush began in earnest when gold was found at Winnecke's Depot, fifty miles north-east of the telegraph station.

As I've said, the only road to the north passed through the station. Along it, in the next few weeks and months, there travelled a weird procession of men and materials.

Gold was then a magic word, much more so than it is today. A few fabulous fortunes had been made elsewhere in Australia, at Bendigo and Ballarat and Bathurst. At Beechworth in Victoria three million ounces were mined in fourteen years. In 1855 an aspiring politician named Cameron rode his horse through the town, drawing attention to himself by the fact that the horse was shod with golden shoes. Thousands of prospectors were flocking to Western Australia where great nuggets of gold were to be picked up in the bush and even in the streets of burgeoning towns. At Coolgardie, years later, the Golden Eagle nugget was found to be worth £6,000. A mere trinket...for twenty years later Brown's Eldorado nugget of 2,000 ounces netted £43,000.

Paddy Hannan, Tom Flanagan and Dan Shea found gold at Kalgoorlie in 1893, only nine years before the time of which I speak. In a single week fourteen hundred eager miners, with gold in their eyes, arrived on the field from the four corners and by 1905 the city had a population of 200,000. Today it is 21,000. The Golden Mile, however, is still Australia's biggest gold mining centre, having produced gold worth more than £200 million.

This was the climate in Australia when the word went out to the world, in telegrams sent by my father and his operators, that gold had been found at Winnecke.

And then, miraculously, the invasion began. There were men in buggies, drays, wagons, sulkies, and on horseback. There were men with packhorses and others humping their blueys; there were even men who pushed handcarts carrying their belongings all the way from Oodnadatta—and if that wasn't the ultimate in doing it the hard way I'd like to know what was.

Alice Springs was transformed almost overnight. The population doubled and then trebled. Whereas we usually saw a new face once a month, sometimes only once in three months, we now had more than we could readily identify.

"Gold near Alice Springs!" the newspapers had announced—

and the same day men who had been heading east or west across the continent turned their faces to the north. Some arrived surprisingly quickly, as men do to any new goldfield, hoping to be first to uncover the nuggets that would put them in clover for the rest of their lives.

As with gold strikes everywhere, the miners were followed by stock exchange manipulators who did their digging fifty miles from Winnecke within immediate reach of the telegraph to Adelaide. Some were honest and some were not, and I wouldn't be surprised if those who were not were the only ones to make any money. They spent endless hours at the station, waiting day after day for telegrams giving them the latest prices and information, and sending their "buy" and "sell" orders on receipt of encouraging or discouraging news from the field.

Our quiet haven became a trading post for sharpies always on the alert for good tips from the "track" at Winnecke. A great many who came to Alice Springs and traded on the Adelaide stock exchange never went near the mines. They created an atmosphere of excitement—of gold-rush fever—that was infectious and, incredibly, even my cautious mother succumbed to it. Not even she was immune to the blandishments of two mining promoters who were entertained in our home and enthused about the prospects of their particular hole in the ground to such an extent that she invested some of her precious savings—quite blindly, on nothing better than the say-so of two men who had everything to gain and nothing to lose.

The run she got for her money lasted just two days. It was then discovered, as might have been predicted, that the promising vein had petered out. Mother lost everything she had invested, but the promoters sold in time.

Shrewd gentlemen of that kind soon lost their popularity around Alice Springs and ceased to be received with anything more than polite formality. They were anathema to the genuine bushmen, especially to Tom Hanley. He was scandalized on hearing that mother had lost her savings and took every opportunity to openly insult the promoters concerned.

He called through the kitchen door one day as a promoter approached, "Are you there, Mrs Bradshaw?"

When mother answered, Tom shouted in the most scathing tones, "Here comes one of your robbers now"

Of course mother was horrified. "Oh, Mister Hanley," she said, "you mustn't say that. He didn't mention investing, you know; it was my own idea entirely."

"Aw!" Tom said disgustedly. "Fancy anyone accepting your hospitality and treating you like that. Robbers, that's what they are, and nothing else!" He seemed ready to strike the man.

And still the prospectors came!

For the rest of that year and throughout 1903 there were new arrivals every week. Hope is said to spring eternal in the human breast, but I wonder where their energy sprang from. They were undeterred by the terrible summer, riding and tramping through the sand, fortified by the artificial rainbow they could see at the end of the trail. Like most rainbows, this one disappeared almost as quickly as it came.

Some of the men arrived in shocking condition. My father's diary for 27th January 1903 records the gift of flour to a group of destitute swagmen who arrived on foot from Oodnadatta. Those who have driven through Central Australia in summer will know what these men suffered as they passed through a living hell. It would have been possible for them to walk only in the early morning and late evening hours; to have walked during the day would assuredly have led to their deaths from dehydration. Even now I am amazed at the courage and endurance of the men who got through and often wonder how many perished and lie in nameless graves in the desert, their bleached bones covered by the drifting sand.

Communications between Alice Springs and Winnecke were primitive for the first year or so...well, for the entire life of the field. Telegrams arriving daily at Alice Springs had to be sent fifty miles by messengers, generally aborigines, who walked both ways in four or five days. The diary for 10th January 1903 reads:

"Aboriginal took telegrams to Winnecke, returned 15th. Another left for Winnecke before return of the first."

It must have occurred to my father that it was high time Winnecke had its own post office. The mail and telegraph traffic had increased to the stage at which it represented a major part of the Alice Springs business. He went to Winnecke by buggy on 13th March, presumably to investigate the need for a post office and report to the authorities on it. But government departments were apparently as slow with their replies in those days as they are today, for it wasn't until six months later, on 3rd September, that the Winnecke post office was opened.

Camel teams arrived frequently with loads for the goldfields at Arltunga and Winnecke. Geologists came too, the experts who would finally determine whether the fields were likely to warrant exploitation by big companies. One of them was the government geologist Mr H. Y. L. ("Geology") Brown who travelled by camel throughout Central Australia in those early years.

Two years passed from the arrival of the first prospectors before I was able to visit Winnecke, but I eventually went there in style—driven in the buggy by Harry Kunoth and with the governess, Miss Mabel Taylor, as companion. We stayed for a few days with the manager of the crushing battery and his wife, Mr and Mrs George Lines.

The road through the hills was unbelievably rough and we were constantly in danger of being thrown out of the buggy. A trace broke and a storm came up. We got off the track several times and were thankful for a haven at Bond Springs station on the first night. The station handyman prepared a guest room across one end of the large stonepaved kitchen. Hessian was stretched over bush timber and wire, and behind it were two bunks made of bagging laced over saplings. They were very comfortable beds but so narrow that I had to climb out to turn over.

These bush-made beds were the rule rather than the exception throughout the Centre in the early days. Most station workers had bunks of bullock hide stretched tight as a drum over a sturdy frame. They had a shelf at the head for a candle or lantern. What more could a man want, especially as they were extremely cool to sleep on? The answer, of course, is that today a man could want inner springs and a fan or an air-conditioned room.

I found Winnecke a calico village, a straggling land of tents and bough shelters. George Lines and his wife lived in two big square tents connected by a breezeway and insulated from the sun by brush walls and a rubberoid roof. This material was also used for the floor. There were deck chairs and improvised furniture, all of it quite comfortable. They even had a small portable organ used for sing-songs in the evening. My diary complains that it was pitched a little too high for the songs I sang and for "Juanita," which I sang as a duet with Mr Lines. No television, no radio, no theatre, no cinema...and yet we had simple fun that kept us very happy.

Whether the miners were happy in their crude humpies is open to question. I'm sure their happiness wasn't dependent on their living conditions but on the nuggets they'd found and the pennyweights they'd dollied.

It is one of the whims of nature that she has generally put mineral deposits in inhospitable corners of the globe —the Yukon, the South African desert, Siberia, and even Kalgoorlie and Coolgardie, which were a long way from anywhere when found. The old girl was running true to form by arranging that gold would be found at Winnecke, and later Tennant Creek.

Like mining fields everywhere—at least until Rum Jungle and Mary Kathleen were born—Winnecke had an atmosphere of ugly impermanence. It was a shanty town which could well have disappeared in the first duststorm. Only the battery had a permanent look about it. How it was hauled there from Oodnadatta, along the incredibly rough trail, boulder strewn and pitted with washaways and gutters, I have no idea. It must have been a colossal undertaking requiring ingenuity and courage. Photographs show that the boiler firing the steam-driven machinery must have weighed many tons. The chimney was thirty feet high. Then there was the ten-head battery itself, weighing many more tons. It all came in wagons from Oodnadatta. The convoy which brought it was held up for six weeks by a breakdown before being able to cross the Finke River. What men they were!

One of my first memories of strident noise is of that gold battery working at Winnecke, with the great crunching clangour reverberating between the walls of the rocky hills. I remember being shown over one of the mines, the Golden Goose, which unfortunately turned out, like the rest of them, to be more goose than golden. I drove to a prospector's camp in a deep gully and there watched alluvial gold being washed by a man who'd walked from Oodnadatta for the privilege of seeing a few colours of gold.

My strongest memory is of Saturday-night shopping in Winnecke village. The miners and prospectors worked all day every day and would have worked at night, too, if there'd been light. As they couldn't, they reserved Saturday night for shopping at the motley of tent-stores and bag-emporiums, perhaps rounding off the evening's entertainment with a visit to Winnecke Hotel, a post-and-rail structure surmounted by a roof of spinifex. How it escaped being set on fire when the rowdy element took over was always a mystery.

On his shopping round each of the prospectors had a long bolster-like calico bag slung over his shoulder in which he carried everything—flour, tea, sugar, rice—and somehow, with a series of knots, prevented one from becoming mixed with the other. The miner would go to a grocery tent and order his week's ration of flour. That would be tipped into the calico bag, which was then knotted securely above it, and the sugar tipped in; it was knotted again, and the process repeated for the tea and the rice until the bag bulged in varying shapes according to the quantity of separate commodities. I often wondered if the miners, having returned home from the hotel, didn't get the sugar mixed with the rice and the tea with the flour. I'm not sure that it's an idea I would recommend to today's housewives.

Nevertheless, it was a colourful scene. There were no street lights, of course, so each of the miners carried a hurricane lantern. These bobbed around like glow-worms as men from all over Australia, as well as Afghans and Chinese, went moodily about their business; most of them, I'm sure, thought of little else but getting back to the holes in the ground which would eventually prove to be their Eldorados.

By day, Winnecke had some of the appearance of a wild-west shanty town—but that description probably flatters it. Yet men and women lived there for four years, making their homes in a corner of the Australian bush that has long since been forgotten.

Early on the morning we were leaving I was sent to buy a tin of fruit from a shed-store run by an Afghan. After knocking on the closed front door without getting an answer I walked around to the back. And there I came upon one of those embarrassing situations that make you feel like an intruder. The faithful soul was on his prayer mat, kneeling and bowing towards the rising sun and presumably Mecca, quite oblivious of the knocking and the interruption I had caused. So I backed silently away, as though I'd committed sacrilege, and left him to his communion with the Prophet. He lost a sale, and for an Afghan trader to do that is proof of his piety.

In July 1903 there was an outbreak of typhoid fever which caused several deaths on the goldfield. Sanitary conditions were such that there was grave danger of an epidemic sweeping Central Australia, with possible fearful consequences if it got among the natives. An appeal was sent south for a doctor. To save the time necessary to bring one from Adelaide, Dr H. W. Shanahan came from Marree with a chemist, Mr Bishop. They must have driven all day and half the night from Oodnadatta because, with only a pair of Timor ponies to pull their buggy across gibbers and sandhills, they reached us in seven days. This was a truly wonderful feat, and a record for the trip at that time.

My father's medical diary shows that he subsequently consulted Dr Shanahan by telegram on several occasions. When the outbreak of typhoid subsided and the doctor departed he left with us a quantity of the best drugs then available. These are also listed in the diary and include digitalis and belladonna.

Less than two years after my original visit I went to Winnecke again with my father. It must have been simply for the drive, or to have a look around, for by then Winnecke wasn't even a ghost town. Except for the big battery standing alone, silent and rusty, the scrub already enfolding it, there wasn't a single reminder that this had once been an industrious if not prosperous mining centre.

I was astonished by the utter desolation of the place. I wondered if I had dreamt that there had ever been a street with several stores, an hotel, and a number of houses. They had disappeared as completely as if picked up in a whirlwind and scattered across the near-by Simpson Desert.

What had happened so suddenly to the men moving over the hills like busy ants at their nests?

What had happened to the horses and buggies, to the Afghans and their strings of camels?

What had silenced the clatter of the ten stampers in the battery, the noise that could be heard for miles and obliterated all other sound?

They had all gone back to where they came from, cashing their colours for a grub-stake to see them through and, for those who were tired or aged, a ride on the coach to Oodnadatta. The song of birds in the mulga, the cark of crows and hawks come to scavenge on the tips, the wail of dingoes and the rustle of trees disturbed by willy-willies—these had returned to claim their rightful places in the natural orchestra that had been lost in the hiss of steam, the grind of wheels, and the stamp of the crusher.

In the gullies farther out there may still have been one or two optimistic fossickers, their hearts less faint, their courage higher, or their stupidity greater than those of the men who had gone. Otherwise there wasn't a sound or a movement or any indication of human life to suggest that this had once been the site of men's hopes.

The ground where the houses once stood had returned to its virgin state. The government battery which George Lines ran had given its answer in the amalgamation pots.

The answer was No or Not Enough.

And under the stampers which battered their ore to powder there died the dreams that had kept men going with their picks and hammers and tappers.

My father and I turned from Winnecke as from a cemetery, for here lay the dreams of men who had laboured as few before them.

But photographs of the hotel, of the battery, and of the house occupied by George Lines and his wife have survived. These show that Alice Springs, instead of being a tourist town, might today have been the pretty neighbour of a Central Australian Kalgoorlie.

In September 1904, after five years on the station, my mother decided that she must have a holiday in the south.

She longed to see her parents and family, her old friends in Adelaide, and, not least, the sea.

For five years she had hankered for a breath of salt air. Having been born at sea and having spent most of her life beside it, I can understand that she was running out of patience with the aridity of the Centre, the spinifex, the duststorms, the summer heat, the isolation, the limited companionship, and the constant gamble with the continued good health of her growing children. Like all those early pioneers, she must have dreaded the thought of serious illness. Anyway, five years seemed a reasonable time to have spent in Alice Springs without a holiday. And so the preparations began, and the excitement mounted, to be capped with the terse entry in my father's diary:

Sept. 12: Mrs. B. and family left for O.D.

How like him to have referred to his wife as "Mrs B." But that was my father all right—courteous, affectionate, and attentive, but reticent and formal in the extreme. The "O.D." was telegraph code for Oodnadatta, as "A.G." was for Alice Springs and "B.K." for Barrow Creek.

The four Bradshaw children then old enough to attend school were overjoyed at the prospect of a long holiday. For almost a year we'd been under the thumb of an experienced teacher, Mrs Louisa Cornock, a widow who had come to us from Adelaide. Our previous governesses had been pleasant and easy-going but academically unqualified. The result must have been obvious in the standard of our knowledge, for Mrs Cornock was frankly horrified, and said so. Efficiency in the schoolroom is not the most endearing trait in any teacher as far as her pupils are concerned; invariably, they react more sympathetically to the principle of *laissez-faire*. But if Mrs Cornock was nothing else she was efficient, and we were on the receiving end.

As children do, we looked on her as an old woman; she was older than my mother, who was still in her thirties, but she wouldn't have been much more than forty-five. Whatever her age, however, when she spoke we jumped to it. We were worked as we'd never been worked before. Saturday mornings had been a free period with other governesses, but with Mrs Cornock we went to our lessons.

Our ultimate grievance with her was that we couldn't enjoy the drive when we went on picnics, as we frequently did; those of us unlucky enough to be sitting in the buggy with her didn't have a chance to chatter about the scenery, the kangaroos, the emus, the aborigines, the sand on the wheels, the horses, or any other things that are important to a child's mind when out-of-doors and on an errand of pleasure; instead we were given mental arithmetic and repetitive tables.

"Consie, eight times nine please?"

"Jack, what is the sum of fourteen and seventeen?"

Is it any wonder that during this period I made a point of always riding to the picnics. And how glad I was that Mrs Cornock couldn't ride, and could not therefore come within spelling distance or history distance of me. I made sure that my horse never approached within easy earshot of the buggy.

To us, Mrs Cornock was straitlaced, but that was apparently a childish impression. She affected others differently. Charlie Tomlin, one of the Barrow Creek linemen, had met her while visiting Alice Springs and became an ardent admirer. Les Spicer remembers that on one occasion when the stationmasters were using the private telephones for a Sunday gossip Mrs Cornock was persuaded to speak to another operator at Barrow Creek. Knowing the background of faint romance, he couldn't let that opportunity pass.

"Charlie!" he shouted across the station compound. "Come quickly! Mrs Cornock is on the telephone and wants to speak to you."

Charlie Tomlin, aged about sixty, disappeared in a terrible dither. When he hadn't returned in a few moments one of the men went to search for him. Poor Charlie, unaccustomed to telephones, was found in a frenzy in his room; his clothes were strewn everywhere and he was trying to get into his "down-south" suit, with an appropriate collar and tie. He was determined that while speaking to Mrs Cornock he would be correctly dressed; he was equally determined not to let her "see" him, or ever suspect that while he spoke to her he was dressed in a pair of pyjamas, which served as summer dress for the men on Tennant Creek and Barrow Creek stations. Having been made by the operators themselves, they were scarcely Savile Row quality. Even if the lady was 170 miles away, I thought it was a nice gesture for Charlie to make. There'd have been more point to it, of course, if we'd then had the television phones I'm told are now on the way.

The prospect of a holiday pleased us immensely, and not only because we would be free of the schoolroom for several months. But what a vast amount of planning and preparation it meant for my mother.

Everything had to be thought out months in advance. She couldn't expect to get what she wanted around the corner at the nearest emporium, for there wasn't one. The township stores carried a meagre stock of clothes, and nothing for girls, so she had to write to Adelaide for samples of dress materials and wait six weeks before they came. Having made her selection and mailed her order, there was then another six weeks' wait for the goods. Three months had passed before, at last, she could spread her paper patterns and begin cutting out, trying on, and sewing. It was an endless business and if for that reason only I'm sure she needed the holiday at the end of it. Fortunately one of the men, aware of her monumental labour, cleverly attached a foot treadle to the hand-operated sewing machine. That was a great help.

Someone else's inspiration turned out a dismal failure. This was a long round canvas bag referred to elegantly as "the valise" and intended to be a convenient carry-all to stow away under the buggy seats. But like a soldier's kitbag it was the most aggravating, temper provoking, thoroughly detestable contraption ever invented. It opened only at one end and, always, the wanted article was at the other. You scrabbled through everything, becoming increasingly irritable, until you were forced to empty the entire bag on the floor or the ground and then push everything back. I know just how soldiers felt about those huge sausage-like kitbags inflicted on them during the wars.

A trunkful of clothes that the six of us would need on the three-day train journey was sent by camels to Oodnadatta, and another was sent straight through to Adelaide to be ready for us on arrival there.

All our oldest clothes were put aside to wear on the track and then be thrown away. Many a pair of patched knickers, many a torn shirt or frock was left to decorate the scrub at our overnight camps. If anyone had really been interested, our trail from Alice Springs to Oodnadatta could have been followed exactly by the clothes we discarded.

One of my former governesses, Miss Elsie Conigrave, who had married one of the operators, Alec McFeat, travelled with us. We also took Vernon, the small son of Mr and Mrs Charles South, who had taken over the Stuart Arms Hotel in Alice Springs. The boy was going to Adelaide for treatment to his eyes. And there was Mrs Cornock.

Harry Kunoth drove the big buggy with its team of five splendid horses. The buckboard came along behind with spare driving horses, packhorses, and two aboriginal assistants. When I look at old photographs of the loaded buggy and realize that we travelled in it for a fortnight in each direction I am amazed that we thought so little of the trip. At first it was an adventure; subsequently it was just a bore, something to be got over as quickly as possible.

We kept an anxious eye on the sky, for neither the buggy nor the buckboard had a hood. From the first day the weather was hot, sultry, and ominous; although rain might not fall for several years, the desert can be a terror when it does, especially during the infrequent equinoctial storms. We also had to face the possibility of the horses bogging if the storm broke; there could be long delays which would seriously embarrass our food position. Perhaps we'd have to live off the land and eat lizards, rats, and dingoes like the nomadic tribesmen. I'm sure I'd have starved rather than do so, yet I'm told that true starvation is a great destroyer of scruples.

On reflection I realize what a tremendous responsibility the journey must have been for mother in her department and Harry Kunoth in his. Twelve white people and three aborigines had to be fed three times a day for a fortnight; except for the stores at Horseshoe Bend and Blood's Creek there wasn't a place on the track where supplies could be replenished.

There was no butcher's shop, yet we must have obtained fresh meat from one of the stations we passed because I clearly remember Harry grilling steak for a dawn breakfast. At that moment mother was still busy packing our overnight clothes and Harry, anxious to get a few miles under the wheels before the sun was too high, gave us our food. Thick slices of steak were wedged between even thicker slices of bread and eaten with the fingers; as far as Harry was concerned, three-year-olds should be able to manage that as well as grown-ups. My sister Edna, who had been born in Alice Springs, was not yet three; she eyed her enormous sandwich from all angles, perplexed at how to attack it but, like any small child in the open air, ravenously hungry and wanting to eat.

"Harry, Harry, I can't get my mouth a-tween," she complained.

Fortunately mother came from the tent at that moment with her hands free and reduced Edna's sandwich to a more manageable size. I couldn't help because I'd already started on

The crushing battery at Winnecke goldfield was brought in by camels and wagons

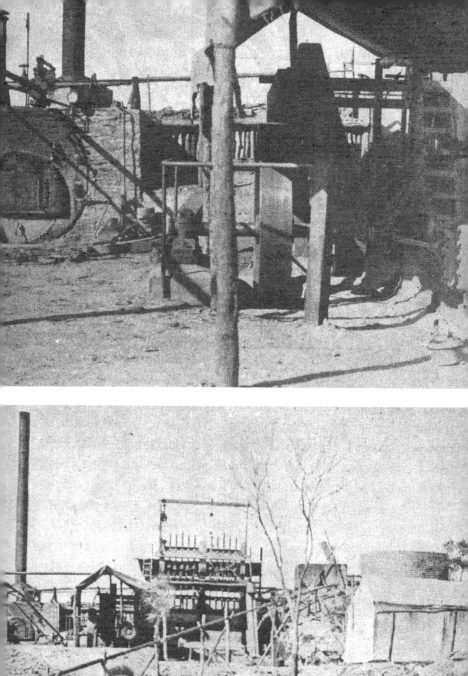
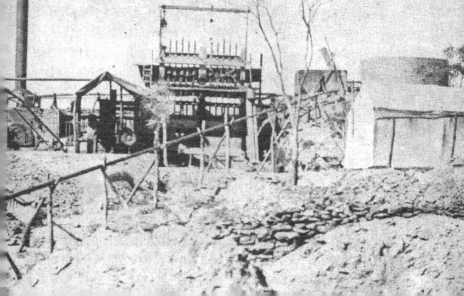

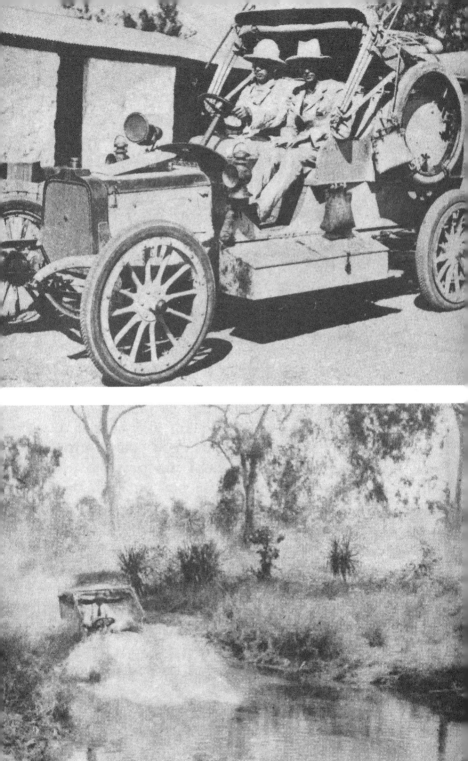

mine and was in midstream, so to speak, with meat, juice, and crumbs all over my face.

The weather continued to be threatening and when we'd gone about half-way to Oodnadatta it finally broke. A thunderstorm came up quickly late one afternoon and we were soon promised a good drenching. There was no sedan hood, no such thing as winding up the windows; I doubt if we even had an umbrella, which wouldn't have helped us much anyway.

The storm came so quickly that the first heavy drops of rain were upon us as Harry swung the team of five horses into lightly timbered country east of the track. Some of us may have wondered, in view of the threat from the skies, why he hadn't done so earlier. We were certainly mystified as he continued to drive in through the scrub with the rest of our circus following. And then, as if by magic, there was a bell tent in a small clearing in the middle of nowhere. I seem to recall Harry saying that it had been left there a year or so earlier by a party of surveyors in order to reduce their load; Harry, superb bushman that he was, knew exactly where to turn off the track to take us there unerringly. I would have passed that spot without knowledge that any kind of shelter was available before reaching Oodnadatta.

We jumped down from the buggies and bundled into the tent while the rain poured down. I have no idea what the aboriginal horseboys or the white drivers did that night except that they must have had a truly miserable time; I do know that ten of us packed like sardines into that old tent with our feet

The first car to cross Australia. Harry Dutton and Murray Aunger at Alice Springs telegraph station, 16 December 1907

My uncle Ernest Allchurch watching Murray Aunger crossing a creek near Darwin
(PHOTO: H. H. DUTTON)

towards the centre pole. It was a night that I'll never forget. Although we were physically exhausted after several days of buggy-riding, sleep didn't come easily. At an unknown hour there was a call in the darkness from my eldest brother, Mort, who was lying nearest the door.

"Mother, my blankets are so wet, and I'm cold," he complained.

And no wonder! When mother lit the hurricane lantern and investigated she found the poor boy was not only wet, but in swirling water. The tent leaked and was now surrounded by a miniature lake. We called the men and they dug trenches to carry the water away. The children on dry ground had to squeeze even closer together to accommodate those lying in water. There were grunts and groans and protests, but they soon subsided when mother took a hand.

It was no use saying, "Oh, mother, Jack's knee is sticking into me," or "Mother, I can't breathe—Consie is squashing me." She spoke firmly and simply, "Not a word from any of you!"

There is an indelible picture of her in my mind recorded at that moment. In the dim light of the lantern I saw her standing among the recumbent forms. She was in sole command of the situation with a bottle of camphor in one hand and a spoon and sugar in the other. To this day I wonder how she found them in that mess. Everyone had to take a dose of camphor sprinkled on sugar as a prophylactic against chill. Not one of us made a fuss; as our turn came we stoically gulped the horrible medicine —and all from the same spoon. When it was Mrs Cornock's turn she made a feeble protest and would have pushed the spoon away. What joy it was to those of us who had been subject to her discipline for months past to hear mother say, "Not a word. Take it." And take it she did, like one of the children.

What a night! Next morning, although the rain had stopped, there were pools of water everywhere, but such is the capacity of desert sand for fluid that we were not delayed by a boggy track. We did have other tribulations though.

That day, Mort, Vernon South, and I travelled in the buckboard with a driver named Paddy McCoy. These horses were particularly tired after the gruelling journey and showed it by lagging behind the big buggy and eventually behind the packhorses as well. They'd been pulling us through sand and over gibbers for ten days or more; there was little feed on the track and they were reaching not only the end of their strength but also their patience.

At the midday dinner camp we met a station worker who offered mother the shelter of his small hut for the night, so we were pressing on to reach it. It must have been built since our first journey north because I couldn't remember passing it before. Finally darkness fell and the horses decided they'd go on strike; normally we camped before dusk and allowed them to graze, but here, towards the end of along haul, they were being asked to pull after dark. Paddy roared and threatened but seemed unable to urge them out of a slow walk. At last, while crossing the sandy bed of a wide creek, they gave up the struggle and stopped altogether.

Paddy became almost demented with rage. Alternately he swore, used the whip, and tried to lead them across, but they wouldn't move another step. In his temper Paddy completely lost his head and flung himself down in the creek-bed...and at that moment, if he was demented, he became suddenly and urgently sane. His ear had come in contact with the sand and he had heard the most ominous of all sounds to a bushman caught in our circumstances. He listened momentarily again, as the aborigines do, then jumped up and yelled:

"Ow, holy heaven, she's in flood and she's coming down...she's coming down."

I could never make up my mind whether Paddy prayed or swore after that. Perhaps there was a little of each, and more of the swearing when we were out of earshot. He seized the whip and began frenziedly lashing the horse which seemed the ringleader of the strike. It was a cruel exhibition and one I did not relish, for the horse had been a faithful servant; nevertheless, this was a dangerous situation and I suppose that Paddy shouldn't be blamed. Stung by the fury of the assaulting whip, the horse reared and kicked. The iron hook on the traces caught in the flesh of its leg and, when the horse moved again, ripped it open. It stood there, trembling and exhausted and perhaps mortally wounded, with blood pouring from a terrible cut. Paddy fairly howled as he unharnessed the poor creature, led it away, and turned it loose. I suppose it died, for we never saw it again.

We had stood helplessly by, watching with horror as Paddy took the doomed animal away. But then I decided that if the creek was really coming down in flood it was time we helped ourselves. Vernon South was quaking with fear, so I hoisted him on my back, told Mort to come with me, and staggered through the darkness and the heavy sand to the far bank. There we waited, not knowing whether we would have to stay there all night or not.

Perhaps the remaining three horses heard the roar of the creek too, or felt its vibrations through their hoofs. In any case, with the strike leader gone, they agreed to move; after a time we could see a subdued Paddy leading them up the bank and through the gloom towards us. We plodded on through the night until we saw lanterns bobbing ahead and met up with a party of aborigines sent back to search for us. It was a great relief, soon afterwards, to reach the tiny hut and see that mother was already sorting out bedding dry enough to be used, and for us to fall in to—for after the experience of the past few hours my nerves were a little frayed and I could think of nothing I wanted more than a warm bed.

Before dropping off to sleep, however, I thought that, of us all, mother would probably be the most thankful when we reached Oodnadatta. Throughout that trip she cared for seven children—her own six and Vernon South—and two women. The former governess, Mrs McFeat, could not be of much help because she was expecting her first baby. She had bravely taken on a buggy ride of more than three hundred miles with a baby almost ready to be born. Then she had to face a three-day train journey of 688 miles to Adelaide. I've no doubt that had the baby been born prematurely on the track my mother would have delivered it safely. Mrs Cornock, although most efficient and a bit of an ogre in the schoolroom, was utterly helpless in the practical business of organizing, feeding, and bedding down a large family; as I've said, mother at one stage had to look after her, too.

As we arrived in darkness we hadn't noticed that near-by Hamilton Bore gushed piping hot water from its artesian flow hundreds of feet below. But we saw it next morning, steaming into troughs, ready-made for baths and laundry. Mother took the opportunity of having local aboriginal women wash our muddy clothes, so that when we started on the trail again we had a valise crammed with clean dresses.

By that time the Alberga River was in flood. We had to cross it that day if we were to catch the fortnightly train from Oodnadatta.

After years of Central Australian dust I thought the flowing Alberga, a hundred yards wide, was a magnificent sight. But I don't think my mother would have been so glad to see it, knowing that somehow seven children, three women, and assorted men and horses had to get across. Nor would she have been fortified by the sight of gum trees obviously feet-deep in the centre of the stream, and the wide expanse of rushing water heavy with debris as it swirled past.

But Harry Kunoth had fought worse battles and been in tighter corners. He took command like a good general directing amphibious troops, giving explicit orders and gaining the confidence of us all—at least of those of us who could swim.

Not having seen enough water to swim in for many years, few of us could.

The aboriginal horseboys were sent through first to select the best track. When their horses swam they knew that way was too deep for the buggy and buckboard, and so they tried again, and again, until they were satisfied about the shallowest crossing. They were followed by the spare harness horses and the pack horses, all of which got through safely. Next came the heavy five-horse buggy. What a good thing it was so high, I thought, and that Harry Kunoth was such an expert horseman. As I watched my mother, the two other women, and brothers and sisters go into the stream with him, I might have been excused if I'd felt a little fear; but I didn't, because I had complete faith in his horsemanship and his knowledge of the bush. On reflection, it seems that during those years we often put our lives in the hands of such practical men as Harry.

We watched the water swirl up to the horses' hocks, to their flanks, and then the bow-wave they made with their barrel-chests. Sometimes it seemed that the water would reach their withers, and then they would swim and the buggy would float downstream—but that didn't happen. Harry flicked his whip if a horse hesitated. This was a moment for firm control and he showed those wonderful animals who was boss. He kept them moving when it seemed that they would struggle and begin to swim. If they'd had toes I would say that in the middle of the Alberga they were on tiptoes. But at last they were across and then it was our turn.

Mort and I, the two eldest children, had been left behind to drive with Paddy. Almost at once we were wading out into the stream. The buckboard was much lower than the buggy and water rushed through it, soaking the stores and forcing us all to stand on the seat to keep our feet dry. Two of the smaller horses began to swim, but the others didn't lose their footing and dragged them through. We were given a small cheer—

and I'm sure mother gave a silent prayer—as we got through the deepest part and the horses began showing more of their flanks above water and finally pulled us to dry land.

Our horses were now so knocked up that fresh ones were sent out from Oodnadatta to pull us over the last few miles of the journey. How the message got so far ahead of us for horses to be sent back in time I was never able to discover, and now there is nobody left to tell me. The fresh horses were harnessed to the big buggy and the buckboard and our tired animals from Alice Springs given a well-earned rest. They could come along with us quietly, grazing on what little feed they could find without having the driver berate them, and trying to recoup their strength for the return trip, whenever that might be.

Yet it was the extra pace that the new teams gave us that led to an accident which might have been fatal and, as it was, was serious enough. Soon after we resumed the journey, my mother, with Edna in her arms, leaned forward on the high front seat of the buggy to admire the skittish team. It was thrilling to be moving at such a good speed again—about six miles an hour—after the snail's pace of the past few days, and we were all in good spirits. As my mother was leaning forward the wheel struck a gutter. The buggy lurched, mother was tossed out of her seat, and was sent flying over the dashboard in front right under the hoofs of the horses. As she fell she instinctively threw Edna, who fell unhurt in the sand, and mercifully the horses didn't kick or trample mother. But it was a very close call.

We saw the commotion, the shouts, and the sudden stopping from our buckboard behind. By the time we drew level mother had picked herself up and she and Harry Kunoth were acting like the leading man and lady in a heavy melodrama, as well they might.

"Oh Harry...Harry...Harry!" she said, half gasping, half weeping, clinging to him in her distress and aware that she could easily have been killed.

One of Harry's big hands was beating a comforting tattoo on her shoulders, although I wouldn't be surprised if he was embarrassed.

"Never mind, Missus; never mind, Missus; never mind, Missus," he repeated, as though it was part of a theme song. Edna, yelling her head off, had been rescued from bushes at the side of the track. We knew at once from the volume of her wails that she was unhurt except for shock and a wounded pride.

So we went on our way—but there were bruises on my mother's knees for months afterwards. They were purple and green and blue, and in later years she had a great deal of trouble with them.

Well, there was Oodnadatta at last, and our boarding house, and how glad we were to see it, and to know that henceforth we would be in the comfort of a railway carriage until we reached Adelaide and began our romp on the beaches and in the parks and visited the friends we hadn't seen for five years. Now the excitement of the holiday began to affect me; for a teenage girl there were so many things I wanted to do, and would do, because we were to be away for about nine months and there would be plenty of time.

But first we all needed a bath after being a fortnight without one on the track. And how we needed it, our bodies coated with grime and dust and sweat. I can't say whether there was a conventional bathroom at our boarding house. I rather doubt it. In any case, mother had a better idea. One of the lubras filled two large tubs with warm water. In one the children in turn were soaped and scrubbed, in the other they were rinsed, just as though they were dirty clothes.

And that night, after a fortnight on the hard ground, we

slept in beds, real beds with mattresses; and though that was long before the day of innersprings, the sheer luxury of the sleep I had in that humble Oodnadatta boarding house has remained one of the strongest memories of my life.

CHAPTER ELEVEN

THE JOYS OF REVELATION

NEXT MORNING THE YOUNGER MEMBERS OF THE Bradshaw family were beside themselves with excitement at the prospect of riding in a train. Edna and Donnell had never seen one, of course, and Jack and Consie were too young when we went north to remember anything about that trip. And, quite frankly, after depending on horses and buggies for five years, Mort and I were also thrilled that we were to travel in style...well, anyway, the best style then being offered by the South Australian Railways Department. How times change! How many children today have never ridden in a train— probably only those who regard trains as declasse. For many, the novelty has worn off flying in aeroplanes. But for us, on that late September morning in 1904, the steam train standing at Oodnadatta station represented the last word in speed, comfort, and modernity.

I remember that Edna and Donnell were utterly fascinated and temporarily quite speechless as we climbed up the steps and took our seats which faced each other along the length of the carriage. Some of those carriages have survived to this day and are used as a kind of lower Second Class accommodation for aborigines. They are commonly known as Dog Boxes, and

I've no doubt that by present standards they are, but to us they were simply splendid.

Donnell, Jack, and Vernon South sat in a row on the edge of the seat, their eyes wide with wonder. As the train began to move, so smoothly that it was almost imperceptible, they looked first at one another, then out the windows and saw the ground and the telegraph poles passing by.

When we had gathered speed and were travelling at about thirty miles an hour, Jack made a discovery that kept him talking about it constantly.

"No bumps. No bumps," he repeated, as though that was the most marvellous thing to have happened in his young life. Having just spent a fortnight in the buggy I could well understand it.

Once they were used to the rhythmical motion they set out to explore the carriage and all its embellishments, and came up with some rather astonishing observations.

"I say," Jack said, "five pounds seems an awful lot just for spitting."

He had carefully read the notice which threatened penalties for various offences, from leaving the train while it was in motion to pulling the communication cord—although I can't remember that our train had such a refinement.

The miles sped painlessly by although not without pain for some, as mother's knees were already troubling her. Fortunately her long dresses hid the unsightly bruises, and planning for the arrival in Adelaide kept her occupied.

That night we stayed at the hotel at Marree, then still known as Hergott Springs. We had travelled more than two hundred miles around the western shore of Lake Eyre, through William Creek and Edward Creek, in a single day! As I write Donald Campbell's Bluebird is being tested on Lake Eyre. It has already travelled at 352 miles an hour and is expected to exceed 400 m.p.h. at any moment. Well, that seems fast by comparison with our humble two hundred miles in a day, but we had been accustomed to a daily maximum of forty.

At the hotel we made the acquaintance of what was to us one of the most marvellous inventions of that age—humble beef sausages. Marree was, and still is, a small village, so I doubt that the dining room boasted a menu. Our meal was simply put in front of us by the proprietor's wife and we ate it or left it as we pleased.

I remember that we had to ask our mother what it was we'd been given—those long oblong shapes of meat, covered in rich gravy, that none of the children had ever seen. I was then thirteen, but I couldn't remember having eaten sausages. And certainly not in Alice Springs, where our thrice-daily meal of meat had been roast, corned, cold, or minced. It seems a small thing to have remained in my memory for so long, but those sausages represented the first real variety in our food for five years and they made quite an impression. The boys decided they could live on them for ever.

Next morning we waited expectantly in the dining-room for breakfast to be served, all of us hoping that we would again get sausages. But not a soul appeared. There were ten of us, plus a few other train passengers, and we thought at first that the unusually large crowd might have delayed the cook. Still nothing happened, and when train time was so near that we either ate then or not at all, mother took matters into her own hands.

"Well," she announced, "I'm going to stir things up," and disappeared in the direction of the kitchen.

Marree competes with Marble Bar as one of Australia's hottest places. The climate in summer is fearful, and days when the thermometer remains below 110 degrees are considered cool. Comparatively, they are. And although that was a September morning, with a pleasant breeze blowing, my mother found the temperature in the kitchen had reached boiling point. The proprietor and his wife were in the midst of such a ding-dong, no-holds-barred row that they had forgotten the customers and took no notice whatever when she walked in.

She must have been terribly embarrassed and hesitated a few moments, wondering whether or not to withdraw. Then she saw that the breakfast was sizzling on the stove, as piping hot as the argument, which showed no sign of abating, so she simply helped herself to ten platefuls of food and carried them back to the dining-room in relays for her hungry brood.

Several men, still waiting hopefully, said "What a jolly good idea," and followed suit. When we'd finished—alas, no sausages!—we cleared our rooms and managed to get to the station and aboard the train with our luggage. The proprietor and his wife still ignored us; she had forgotten to feed us and he to assist us to the train, which was a normal courtesy that publicans extended to clients in those days. I hope they didn't also forget to collect their money.

Quorn that night, with a population of a few hundred, seemed a vast city. Goodness me, it had footpaths, and several hotels, and many shops, and even street lamps! They reminded me nostalgically of the old lamplighter who had come down Halifax Street in Adelaide at dusk every evening, pedalling his bicycle and stopping beneath each lamp to pull the chain which lit it.

Jack had been less than two years old when we left for Alice Springs and had never seen street lamps. Now he said, "Mother, aren't the people kind to light up the track for us." The use of the word "track" was significant too; until that moment he was unaware that tracks sometimes became roads. The younger ones also had the thrill of spending money for the first time; I remember that one bought a pineapple and another a coconut—and they were assuredly the first of either of those that we'd seen.

At Peterborough we left our carriage for the luxury of one built to broader specifications, for that was then the terminus for the break of gauge. Almost at once mother began to transform us too. Adelaide was only a few hours away. Our relatives would be at Central Station to meet us, and we didn't want to give the impression that during five years in that distant desert we had "gone native."

So one by one we were taken into the little washroom at the end of the carriage to emerge resplendent and shining in new clothes, smiling sheepishly at one another, discomfited in glad-rags that had cost my mother six months of planning and effort. These were the "Adelaide" clothes that had been put aside as each garment was completed, not to be worn until this ultimate moment of our arrival in the city. None of us had imagined, of course, that our dressingroom for this conversion would be the W.C. on a train. It could have been worse. At least it had privacy.

There we sat, stiff as ramrods on the edges of our seats, our hands folded in our laps, containing our fidgets as best we could, trying not to betray the trepidation and the ferment that all country children feel on arrival in a roaring metropolis. Mother could not have known how long it would take her to get seven children and herself ready to face the critical city-slickers, as I remember that she allowed too much time; we had an interminable wait as the train, really travelling now, pulled away from Gawler and took us into a fairyland of gas lamps and trams and buildings fifty feet high and so many people hurrying back and forth that we were utterly bewildered and yearned at once for the peace and quiet of Alice Springs.

And on the platform, among the people there to meet us and our travelling companions, came the last catastrophe of the trip. That horrid valise, bulging to bursting point, played the last mean trick by spitefully opening its seams and allowing its contents to spill across the platform. All the dreadful relics of camping gear and our soiled clothes went tumbling and rolling around people's feet, tripping and confusing them and making them stop and stare at us...the country cousins come to town. Conspicuous among our chattels, needless to say, was an indispensable bedroom utensil not usually rolled along a station platform. That caused everyone to laugh uproariously and an even greater crowd gathered to join in the fun. But for us, trying to look like little ladies and gentlemen in our lovely new clothes, kid gloves and all, it was a terrible moment of mortification and humiliation. We were glad when finally we were bundled into the Glenelg train and whisked away to the furnished house waiting for us there.

It was a large, interesting old house that had been lived in by doctors for many years. Now it was to be our home for almost nine months—months that were filled with new experiences for us all, new sights, new friends, a new school, and the sea.

I remembered the ocean at Glenelg from the days we had spent there before going to Alice Springs, but for the rest of the family it was their first view of the sea. And what a thrill that was!

"What a big waterhole!" Jack said. For a boy who had been brought up in the arid heartland, and had never seen more water than in the flooded Alberga River a few days earlier, that was an understatement.

"Does it get deep in the middle?" Donnell asked. "And look at all the soap on it!" Edna said.

The days and weeks passed in a delirium of youthful pleasure, of sausages and sausages, of different food, of fresh fruit and fresh cream, of grapes and strawberries, of peaches and pears, of the ice-cream man in his little cart, of the post-man calling, of the trains and the trams and the boats and the marvellous endlessness of it all. None of these things were available to us in Alice Springs and while we were there we perhaps didn't miss them; but now we were here and they were here, so we made a point of getting acquainted.

Guy Fawkes Day arrived. We'd never heard of it, so we had no idea what it was, and our mother had to explain about the dreadful Mr Fawkes whose fame had not spread to our humble schoolroom in Central Australia. I remember we tumbled out of bed that November morning and ran into Moseley Street to gaze in wonder at the first guy we'd ever seen, and in awe when told that at night he'd be put on a huge bonfire and burnt. And there'd be crackers and rockets and double-bungers that would have made every Aranda tribesman head for the hills in the belief that malevolent Kadaitcha Men were after them. My father's diary records that on Guy Fawkes Eve, Harry Kunoth returned to Alice Springs. He'd been absent for seven weeks, driving horses for nearly seven hundred miles. And he did it regularly.

Then there was Christmas, to us a magical festival here in the city. Never had we imagined such shops, such toys, such gorgeous decorations, and such crowds.

In Alice Springs, so we'd been told, Father Christmas had a rather special arrangement with mother. After he received our letters he sent the toys on the mail coach because, as Mort had sagely observed, "Santa Claus can't drive up here—his reindeers couldn't get through in this drought." So our presents came weeks in advance and were safely hidden until The Day. We knew that we should never expect the old man to bring them personally; having travelled from Oodnadatta by buggy we realized the distance was altogether too great for a sleigh. What Father Christmas missed the telegraph operators gained. They had a wonderful time every year helping our parents to fill the stockings—first four and later seven—and, like boys everywhere, trying out the mechanical toys.

But here in Adelaide we saw the kindly old gentleman in person; not only that, we went into a big shop and actually spoke to him. That so excited us all that poor mother almost gave up hope of any sleep on Christmas Eve. Each time she cautiously crept to the bedroom door the same head popped up from the pillow, determined to see the wonderful sight of that old gentleman bringing the doll she'd asked for. It wasn't until two o'clock in the morning that she was overcome by sleep and Mrs Santa Claus was able to steal quietly into the room and then climb wearily into her own bed.

And that night, one thousand miles away, my father wrote in his diary: "Mr and Mrs George Lines drove in from Winnecke goldfield to spend Christmas at Alice Springs with me." Well, at least my father wasn't lonely without his family. In fact, he was soon to join us in Adelaide. The diary shows that he left Alice Springs in summer heat on 5th January 1905, and was with us at the beach three weeks later.

Billy Crick, the telegraph station gardener, also came south on leave that summer. He invited mother to meet him in the city for a "day out" which, as it transpired, became something of a free circus for the locals.

They began by taking a ride along Rundle Street in a horse-drawn tram. On alighting, Billy was convinced that he'd been given short change. He might have been a hayseed, he said later, but he wasn't going to let any tram driver do that to him. He and the conductor argued about the fare until, having to keep to schedule, the tram moved on and left Billy and mother standing in the street, with Billy still shouting his head off. Billy managed to attract the first part of a crowd around him by chasing after the tram and continuing to abuse the conductor at each of the stops.

When he tired of that he rejoined mother for a period of window-shopping. Billy was attracted especially by a display of woollen underwear—good, practical, sensible stuff for those times. He held forth on the advantages of each garment, selected what he'd like to wear, and gave the reasons why, to the huge delight of the gathering crowd. Poor mother hadn't the heart to spoil his pleasure by pointing out that all the articles in the window were for women only. She arrived home nervously exhausted after a day which had led from one embarrassment to another, but she said she'd no doubt enjoy the memory of it all in years to come.

Gradually the novelty of the city wore off, in spite of the joys of a summer at the seaside and our addiction to sausages.

After the freedom we'd known at Alice Springs our lives were subject to unaccustomed circumscriptions. Our movements were restricted. We had to catch a train or a tram to go anywhere. There were no horses to ride. The weather was sometimes cold and wet and we had to stay indoors, a restriction that bothered all of us.

The crowds had interested us at first but soon became tiresome. I remember four-year-old Donnell stamping his small foot in exasperation in Rundle Street one day while trying to pull a wheeled toy along the footpath.

"Jolly people!" he exploded. "Why must they always get in my way?"

Perhaps that was how we all felt, secretly a little superior to these poor creatures who had to live every day in a city and compete with thousands of others for their needs. They seemed distracted and discomfited by their ant-like scurrying and we were sorry for them. Few had any idea of the luxury of being able to spread out in hundreds of square miles of vacant country.

And so, as the time for our return drew nearer, we became more than ever ready to get back to our own land, to the joys and tribulations of our Central Australian isolation, to our dear magnificent horses and the freedom to ride out into the unspoilt bush. Nor were we discouraged by the knowledge of the arduous trip ahead before settling down once again at the telegraph station. Familiarity with the long train and buggy ride had certainly not made us contemptuous of what we had to suffer, but at least we knew what to expect.

We assembled at the railway station one winter morning, thankfully without the valise, and with a new governess, Miss Mabel Taylor. She had never been far from the city and must have been a little fearful of the forbidding desert she'd read about and the formidable distance. But she was travelling with people who had "been there," as we frequently insisted, and that may have been a comfort to her.

We were able to initiate her, to tell stories about the places we passed in the train, and even to extol the virtues of our primitive camping arrangements on the track when we were once more reduced to five miles an hour in the buggies.

This was my third crossing of the desert in an open horse-drawn vehicle, and I was just fourteen years old.

My father's diary records that from Oodnadatta to Horse-shoe Bend we averaged 4.7 miles an hour and from there to Alice Springs, through the Depot Sandhills, 3.5 m.p.h. The horses arrived with shoulders chafed from the collar. That wasn't surprising in view of the tremendous pull through the sand. I see that they were treated with a knob of Reckitt's Blue, a pint of kerosene, and unslaked lime! This treatment was continued daily until the sores healed.

My own recollection of the journey is that it was uneventful. Presumably one grows accustomed to anything in time. Uneventful, indeed! I'm sure for someone who had never done the trip it might well have provided the material for a book.

We drove in style through the small township, waving to the local residents who had come to their doors to welcome us back. How good it was to be back, to be home again!

Yes, home...for to all of us Alice Springs had become the home we loved.

The horses found their own way through Middle Park, now in the pastures that were home for them too; they whinnied and shook their heads in answer to the animal greeting from the stockyards, anticipating the long rest they had earned so well, the freedom from collars and hames and traces that they might expect until their strength was fully restored.

The aborigines on the bank of the river "yak-aied" as we came into view and even their dogs barked a welcome. The station staff were all out to meet us, their faces wreathed in broad smiles, all anxious for some chatter and the news from "down south."

But first we had to be inspected and assessed:

"My goodness, look at Edna and Donnell—how they've grown!"

"And Doris, doesn't she look well?"

And we in turn greeted each member of the staff and complimented them on their apparent good health.

The station village, still larger than the township, had grown in our absence. My uncle, Ernest Allchurch, had married Elizabeth Williams, Mrs Meyer's younger sister, at Hermannsburg Lutheran Mission and he and his wife were established in a small log-and-thatch cottage near the vegetable garden, complete with a domestic staff of aborigines—Peter and his wife Mary Ann. That was an added excitement for our return; it meant that we had a married couple living on the station and another house for us to visit.

Shortly after we'd settled down Leslie Spicer was appointed to the staff, arriving by the mail coach in July 1905. Sixty years later we are still firm friends. He lives quite near my home in Adelaide and we see each other frequently to reminisce about old times. He has given me a letter he wrote to his sister immediately after arriving in Alice Springs which gives a good idea, through male eyes, of what mail-coach travel in the outback was like:

> I was quietly eating my breakfast at Oodnadatta when I heard a yell, "Coach is starting!" I grabbed my swag and

Inner courtyard of the old telegraph station

Old telegraph station homestead, now the centre of the reserve

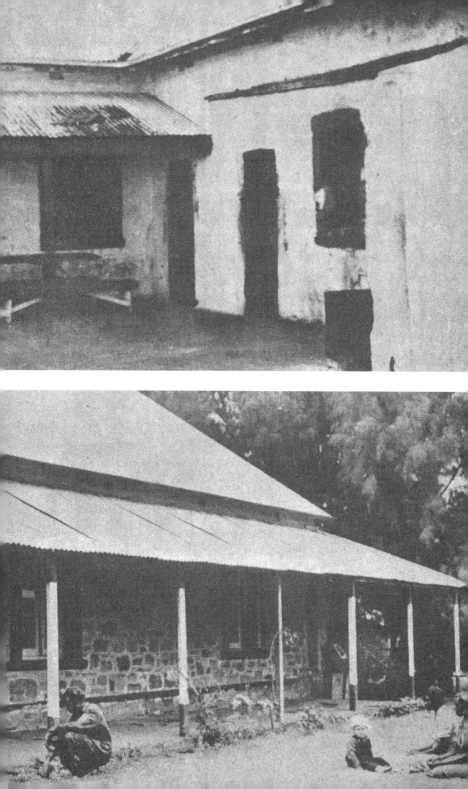

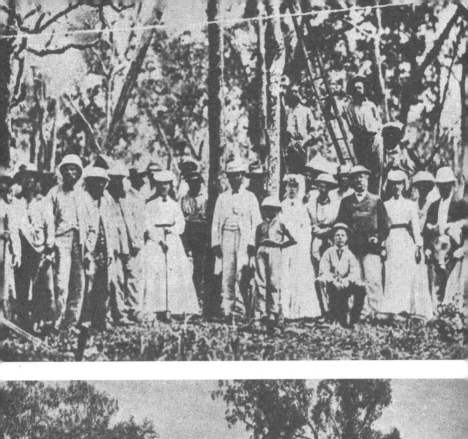

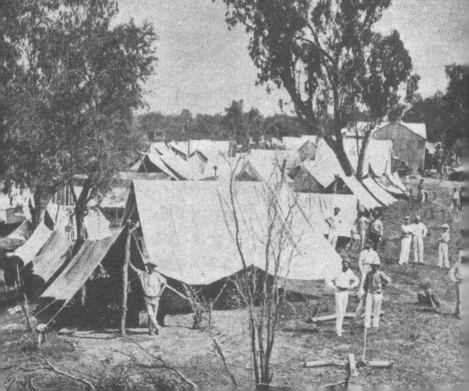

sprinted up the street, but then had to wait two hours for the driver. The coach was a high-seated buggy; here were three of us on the only seat, with another passenger keeping the black boy company on top of the mailbags behind. Harry Tilmouth was driving a five-inhand team with three colts in the lead. The boys had pulled off the hobbles and were hanging on to the horses' heads. As Harry swung his whip and shouted "Let go!" a man rushed up with two bottles of beer as a parting gift. In making a grab for them the driver dropped his nearside rein.

Ben Hur in a chariot race had nothing on us. We rattled over the gibbers at a hand-gallop, around Harry Gepp's store, knocking off only one veranda post and missing the telegraph posts by an eyelash. There were no fences to stop us. We shed the passenger and the native on the mailbags quite early, as well as everything else that could move. Finally one of the others, watching his chance, grabbed a flying rein and hung on till he brought us to a standstill. The beer was saved.

That was the start of twelve days' travelling. Incredibly, we found fish in waterholes around some of the bores— bony bream sometimes weighing up to two pounds. There are also acres of bulrushes, though only a few years ago there was nothing but desert. Don't ask me where the fish and the reeds come from. At Hamilton Bore we met an aboriginal letter carrier. He wore the remains of a singlet, carried a boomerang and two spears in his hands and a mailbag on his head.

Planting the first O.T. dote near Palmerston, 1870
(PHOTO: P.M.G. DEPT.)

Roper River Camp, 1872
(PHOTO: P.M.G. DEPT.)

At Blood's Creek the thing that struck me most was the storekeeper, Old Man Bailes, feeding his five glossy cats on a stool at the table before he attempted to carve a morsel for himself or his guests. Leaving late, the driver managed to break three springs in the buggy when travelling too fast down a stony hill. After that we crept along. At night heavy rain fell and in the morning our horses had gone. The rain had stretched their greenhide hobbles and they had come off. Growing tired of waiting, I walked into Horseshoe Bend and met Mr Sargent. His dogs met me first and obviously didn't recognise me as a cash customer. Rain water must have been scarce for there was a warning over the drinking supply tank:

NOTIS

Enny person drinken this worter will dye
sune as we are gom to poison it next week.

At Horseshoe Bend another driver, Tom Williams, took over Leslie Spicer's coach and his education in bush ways. Tom was as hardy a bushman as ever existed and full of contradictions.

Leslie's letter continues:

The first thing I noticed was his knowledge of Shakespeare, especially anything concerning Falstaff, and it wasn't long before I realised where his strange oaths came from. I admired his fluency and he laughed.

"Yes, I used to read Shakespeare a lot; he taught me to swear," Tom said.

There were some very strange travellers on the track. One of them named "Flash Johnnie" appeared to be a most likeable type, and I asked the driver: "He seems a fine chap, Tom; what's flash about him?

"The cow always carries a toothbrush," Tom said.

Toiling through the Depot Sandhills we hailed an old man walking. Tom offered him a lift but it was declined. I was told his name was Mueller, that he was a brother of the first officer-in-charge of Alice Springs telegraph station; that he was a fine geologist, and had at one time been headmaster of a leading Adelaide school. He had given up many years of life to the search for gold and was on his way then to the field at Aritunga. He carried no blankets, travelling everywhere only with a sugarbag of food and a billycan. Like the blacks, he slept either in a hole in the ground in which he'd previously had a fire or between a circle of small fires.

The weather was wet and cold, the horses in rather poor shape, and the track extremely heavy. At one stage, of which I gladly walked some distance, we covered twenty-two miles in eleven hours. The indomitable driver was far from well but kept saying, "I'll be all right when I reach home." Visualising the place, I expected various comforts, a warm bed and roaring fire. Instead, at his home at Deep Well, we boiled the usual billy in the kitchen and ate the usual salt meat. Tom spread his usual blankets on the cement floor while I preferred the sand outside.

On the last day into Alice Springs a dingo jogged alongside the coach for several miles, about fifty yards distant. Finally it got on Tom's nerves, so he picked up his rifle and shot it. The animal writhed for a moment and Tom half regretfully said, "I shouldn't have done that; there was plenty of room both for him and for me in this country." Tom dismissed another character we met as "Too polite to be honest," and events proved him to be right.

Except for the "wild west" take-off from Oodnadatta I think Leslie's experience would be par for the course on the mail run to Alice Springs, although perhaps his own return journey was stranger still. He walked the entire distance and thinks so little of it that I can't persuade him to discuss it in detail. "Why, I just walked all the way," he says. It was a walk of more than three hundred miles.

Leslie returned south during the first World War to enlist in the army. He was offered a ride from Alice Springs on one of two camels owned by a surveyor, Mr Jack Waldron. The offer was accepted, but before they set out two men asked if they might also accompany the party. One had tuberculosis and was a very sick man; the other was unable to walk any long distance. So Leslie walked—and sometimes outpaced the camels. He, even made a detour to visit Mr and Mrs Alex Ross, who were then at Dalhousie station, several miles off the beaten track. The walk was a pleasant experience, he says, and a useful prelude to army training. Well, everyone to his preference.

Some of our "down south" clothes weren't suitable for wear in the Centre, so there was a grand hand-out to aborigines and to a Chinese family then living in the village. The father, Ah Hong, accepted the gift but with Oriental politeness insisted on making one in return. Some months later an aboriginal messenger arrived from Wallis's; store. He had a small packet and a formally worded letter from Hong written by the manager, George Wilkinson. But there was also a postscript from George: "What Hong really said was, "No-more gibbit big girl, you say gibbit little one." So I missed out on a gold bracelet set with a diamond and rubies, which was kept for my youngest sister, Edna. Together with the faded note from a grateful Chinese, it has remained with her in England for more than twenty years.

The motoring bonnets we'd had in Adelaide were a thrill for the lucky recipients. Goodness knows why we possessed them at all—it certainly wasn't for any motor tours we'd done. They were large cloth caps with a small brim; a "gossamer" was draped over the top and tied coyly under the chin to anchor the hat in place as one whizzed along at a good ten miles an hour. "Queen" Luitchira got my red one, and it completed her ensemble perfectly she was a skinny, ugly old aboriginal woman who usually wore a tattered shirt, with a clay pipe stuck behind her ear.

Our new governess, Mabel Taylor, did an unheard of thing: she made a divided skirt to wear while riding a horse—a long, full, and discreet skirt, to be sure, covering her to the very ankles, but a divided skirt, nevertheless, which would enable her to ride astride instead of side-saddle. Never had a woman been seen in that country riding any other way than side-saddle. Quite a few of the locals were shocked, or made out that they were, by this daring innovation.

But such comforts were not for me. I was still a child when my side-saddle was bought and a horse broken in to get used to my long flapping "habit." My parents were rather staid in such matters and I realized the futility of rebellion, so put up with it as best I could. I loved riding and would suffer any discomfort to enjoy it, but what a silly old English custom to cling to in the Australian bush. The side-saddle, moreover, was extremely uncomfortable for the rider when the horse was either ascending or descending a hill, and it was much worse for the unfortunate animal. Mounting was made awkward and I still feel ashamed when I think of the energy, the strength, and the gallantry needed to hoist me into my saddle, especially as I was a girl of the type frequently described, like a horse, as "upstanding." I envied Miss Taylor and what was then the New Look.

Still, I had the advantage when we played tennis and she had to wear the long heavy skirt and petticoat every woman did as a matter of course. What torture they were, and how impractical; yet a woman was thought to be immodest if she showed an ankle.

Tennis? Yes. After Leslie Spicer's arrival an interest in tennis developed and an earth court was made on the station.

That was considered to be a little anti-social, so later on one was built in the township to give others a chance to join in. Land was bought between Wallis's store and the Stuart Arms Hotel and an earth court finished in 1906. It stood back from the road and was surrounded by shady gums. Dust and all, we enjoyed playing there.

After our game we sometimes went to visit Mrs Alex Ross, who at that time had come in from the bush to live in an old house not far from Wallis's store. These visits were always a joy as she possessed a flair for story-telling. We revelled in her sense of humour and in her simple yet often rib-tickling yarns about the Inland and its people.

During these years my brother Mort and I were enrolled at the Adelaide School of Art and became its most distant pupils. Those lessons were the only help we ever had by correspondence; otherwise, for nine years, we were entirely dependent on the governesses and ourselves. When Mabel Taylor had completed her term and gone back to Adelaide it seemed impossible to get anyone to take her place. So the four other Bradshaw children of school age were taught by me, their sixteen-year-old eldest sister.

I remember one day as I sat with them in the tiny school-room and set their lessons I was overcome by the realization that my own school days were finished. There could be no going back. And thinking of all I had wanted to do I shed the bitter tears of an adolescent girl. Perhaps my reward for what I personally missed lies in the fact that when the time came for the children to attend school "down south" they were able to take their places in the normal classes for their ages. It was gratifying to know that my efforts for more than a year had at least kept them to that standard.

Quite obviously, this situation could not be allowed to continue. For that reason, among others, my parents decided in 1908 that to give the children a chance it was necessary to move back nearer to what some people like to call "civilization"—their word for the teeming cities of mankind.

So once more the planning and the preparation began, the orders for materials were sent on the mail coach. Once more, at the end of three months, my mother had to work overtime at the sewing machine. By now there were seven of us to be made as presentable as possible "for Grandma." Mother, who'd been born at sea, had a high opinion of her own mother's good taste in clothes and every garment was made with the hope of her approval. She was longing to see her mother again and thrilled, too, at the prospect of furnishing a home. So much to think of and to plan! The candles and the hurricane lights burnt late at night.

The family didn't share her enthusiasm about leaving Alice Springs. On the contrary, there were one or two of us who wanted to rebel, and at least refuse to budge unless we could take our horses with us. Our attitude was, "Botheration to Adelaide; we've been there once; we don't want to go again; we want to stay here—at home with the horses." Of course, our opposition and our opinions were futile; a decision had been made by the Master and Mistress of the house and we would do what they said.

If possible, the aborigines were even more upset than we were. They had been treated by my father for nine years with scrupulous fairness. He had shown them mercy in the courts of law where he sat as Special Magistrate, and mercy to the aborigines wasn't always common in the Centre of the early days. On occasions he had punished white people who transgressed the laws of humanity affecting the black people, and that was rare indeed.

"Adnutta...Boss...you no-more bin go-away," they pleaded.

It was no use. We were going, and we were going for ever.

When the aborigines discovered that the children who had been born at Alice Springs were leaving too, they became highly indignant. Apparently it hadn't occurred to them that anyone, white or black, could leave the country of his birth. They still have this idea today. But they were to be disillusioned—Donnell, Edna, and Alan were coming with us, whatever claim the Arandas might have to them.

They came to my father and my mother repeatedly pleading for the right of the children to remain in their ancestral home.

"No good you bin take'im that piccaninnies," they said.

"Him bin grow'up Tonga this place; no good you bin take'im Tonga 'nother country; you leave'im Tonga Aranda."

Our pretty little half-caste nursegirl, Amelia, wept for days when she learnt that we were leaving. She begged and implored mother to take her too. Like all aborigines, she had come to love the children she cared for as though they were her own. I thought her heart would break.

Mother was so disturbed by her grief that she talked it over with my father, but both agreed it would be foolish and no kindness to the girl to take her so far away from her tribe, with little hope of getting back if she once grew homesick, as she inevitably would.

Fifty years later that same nursegirl, then a grey-haired woman with her own family of eight, stayed with me in Adelaide. She had married Harry Kunoth. She still spoke sadly of the parting with the Bradshaw family as though it had been the rock-bottom period of her life.

"Nobody has ever been as kind to me since," she said. "I loved your Mum."

And I knew that she did.

Just before we left, and not before time, workmen arrived from Adelaide to build a gaol in the township. There was no public hall, or any of the other utilities common to most towns, but a gaol...well, that was an essential.

The log cabin gaol at Heavitree Gap police station was certainly a farcical piece of work, but it did seem odd that one of the first substantial buildings the government built in Alice Springs township, as distinct from the telegraph station, was a place for the incarceration of its citizens. In all our years there, I could remember only one white man who had spent any time in prison. He acted as cook for his two warders, one presumably for night duty and the other for day duty. When it was suggested to the warders that they were treating the white prisoner extremely well one of the guards said, "Oh well, it might be our turn next week and Jim might be guarding us." Which is exactly what happened.

As the time for our departure drew near, the townsfolk, who still numbered only a dozen, decided to join with a few from the nearer cattle stations in arranging a farewell for our parents. This was to take the form of a surprise party. Unfortunately one of the men working on the new gaol gave my Uncle Ern a hint of what was afoot and he, being male and unable to keep a secret, passed it on to mother. That poor workman, Danny Marr, was "sent to Coventry" by his mates and was the only soul not at the party.

Mrs Rodda, the wife of one station cook, had been a ventriloquist and still possessed her dolls, Nelson and Wellington. They were slightly the worse for wear, as I remember them, having been bumped on buckboards and camels from Queensland to the Kimberleys and down through Central Australia. But she was the life of the party. She gave such a polished performance in our sitting-room that night that poor old Ah Hong was almost beside himself with astonishment. He dashed to the fireplace and peered up the chimney looking for the hidden voice. He opened cupboards and looked under furniture, quite carried away by the reality of it all and oblivious of everybody. Ah Hong, though he didn't know it, was the star turn of the evening.

Then the day came. There was a sad sense of finality about our going, but the greatest wrench of all was the parting from beloved horses which had carried us hundreds of miles on journeys of enchantment through and beyond the MacDonnell Ranges. I was old enough to realize that, in Adelaide at least, there would be no more riding for me. This was a joy that was difficult to relinquish without a sob, and I'm sure that I sobbed. And, as though they knew it, there was a whinnying from the stockyard as we drove out through the station gates for the last time. The natives came up from their camps and lined the road in mute salute, some standing sadly and with eyes only for the children, others sitting with their heads covered in token of mourning.

Passing through the township we were farewelled by the few permanent residents from the doors of their shops and dwellings, and finally by the men working on the gaol—that symbol of fetters paradoxically set up in an unfettered land. They were the last people I remember seeing in Stuart, as it still was.

We didn't go far before making camp that first night. It was just as well. For while we were preparing our midday meal next day a native, riding hard, arrived from the station with a telegram for father. There was an ominous hush as he read it, a foreboding of bad news, and then he took mother aside and we heard her cry.

He came to us then and said quietly, "Your grandmother died yesterday, just as we left."

This was a crushing disappointment as well as a tragic loss for my mother, especially as my grandmother's death was quite unexpected. There was worse to come: at Charlotte Waters and Oodnadatta we got letters that were heartbreaking…for they were bright letters from a lady who was now dead saying how much she was looking forward to seeing us all again. It was several days later that her son, Uncle Ernest Allchurch, still on his way to Darwin by car with Harry Dutton and Murray Aunger, learnt of her death. He had not seen her for five years.

The old had gone but the new was here...a young family of seven grandchildren waving a last goodbye to Oodnadatta, leaning from the windows of the train for a longing look at the horses until they were out of sight...knowing that this last link with the life and the home we had known in Alice Springs would disappear for ever the moment we had crossed the plain.

After more than sixty years the memories might be expected to come dimly through the joys and sorrows of my own married life, and the birth and care of my own children. Yet they are vivid and detached and sharp, and I know that they will never go away while light remains in my mind ...

...riding through Heavitree Gap and crossing the Todd on a clear calm evening in the Australian heartland, the moonlight shining on the glistening white trunks of ghost gums towering up on the slopes of the ranges...the ghost gums that have become a trade-mark throughout the world for the Namatjiras, the Inkamalas, the Pareroultjas, and the other water-colourists descended from those naked nomads who camped and corroboreed at the bottom of our garden. and mourned when we went away...

...a black stormy evening, with the Todd in swift flood. I was walking home alone from the village, having been left behind through a misunderstanding. And I waited for the next flash of lightning to show me a path among the tumbled rocks on the edge of the swirling water. And through all the turbulence, and above the cymbals of the heavenly music, the mournful call of curlews, rising and falling, as though they, too, were frightened to be alone and expressed my fears. A night for a child to remember...

...looking down from the brow of a hill on the silent, sleeping station below, the roofs shimmering beneath the moon...a haven small but secure among the prehistoric rocks encircling it...

...gazing westward from the MacDonnells into the tangerine sunset, trying to comprehend the thousand miles of desert beyond, empty of known human habitation...

...the memory of just a handful of people brought together in that isolation, utterly dependent on each other for companionship, for help in need, for sharing good and bad, for mingling laughter and sorrow, for learning from the bush a true sense of values.

I am rich in my priceless memories.

Who could forget the spell of the Inland, the relentless country that has to be understood before it can be tamed?

Who could forget the majesty and the beauty brooding in the primeval silence? Not I.

What they call Progress has come to it, and will come increasingly.

And fame, too.

But I love to remember it when it was all ours...in those long ago days when it was our home.

And I like to say now, when asked where I was brought up and educated, "Alice...On The Line."